REVELATIONS OF YOUR SELF-HELP BOOK SECRETS

Neuroscience and Psychology of the Self-Help Literature as it Reveals the Challenge of Understanding Thought Projection Outside Our Human Brain

by
Lancaster Adams

Strategic Book Publishing and Rights Co.

Strategic Book Publishing and Rights Co.
12620 FM 1960, Suite A4-507
Houston, TX 77065
www.sbpra.com

ISBN 978-1-61204-146-9

DEDICATION

This book is dedicated to Cheryl, Ashley, Evan, and Peter

PREFACE

"Remember that not getting what you want
is sometimes a stroke of luck"
—The Dalai Lama

You have picked up this book to see if you can learn if your self-help book's advice is based on fact or fiction. You want to know if you are getting your money's worth, and the results that will flow from your striving. This book is here to help you. Using examples culled from my own life's odyssey, new advances in neurobiology, readings in self-help, and quantum physics, I trust that I can paint a realistic picture for you without boring you with equations, of which this book has none.

In fact, this book has left out all the physics experiments for easier reading. The most you'll get is a line or two about the double-slit experiment. This was the famous experiment that Richard Feynman, the brilliant physicist, used to describe how particles moving through the slits traversed all possible paths, engaged in all possible histories, and could traverse the universe and back, acquiring information along the way. This helped support your self-help book's theories on a universal mind. Do you believe the contention that you can log on to this universal energy field and direct your own future?

It's powerful, fun stuff that this book hopes to sort out for you, but as the Dalai Lama cautioned, be careful what you wish for.

And when the reading gets a little too heavy, a little light-hearted humor is injected.

Even the great mathematical genius Richard Feynman found time to relax, sipping a beer or playing the bongo drums at a local strip club. Dream analysis with all its pitfalls is used as a demonstration of paranormal and metaphysical quandaries.

You will be presented with the vision of your self-help book from the viewpoint of a biological scientist and medical doctor, rather than that of a physicist. In over seventy-five texts and books on quantum physics that I have read and digested for you, it is clear that most physicists think in terms of mathematics, which is not the usual lingua franca of your daily existence. So I have presented some of the tougher material in terms that you and you neighbors can discuss, and come to your own conclusions. It may seem overly simplistic at times, but rest assured the underlying science is still exciting and valid.

At times my critique of the other seventy-five-odd books that I have read on self-help, some of which I still use daily, may seem a little harsh. This is mainly to help you ask your own questions, and think through more clearly what you are getting yourself into as you engross yourself in the self-help book messages. At the end of the book I hope and trust that you come away with a much deeper understanding and explanation of what is really going on. Also, I hope you find much joy and wisdom in some of my favorite quotations, which can serve as useful crutches when challenges appear in your life.

This is, in the final analysis, about you. As of this writing, Halloween is coming up on the calendar. My fervent wish is to sweep away all the hallows or ghosts that clog our minds in the form of unproven superstitions, whilst still retaining rational explanations and wonder for some of the weird occurrences that you undoubtedly can relate to in your own life, and the seemingly miraculous manifestations obtained through applying your self-help book material. Please enjoy!

ACKNOWLEDGEMENTS

This book was written with a review of over 150 books in the fields of time, quantum physics and, of course, self-help books. Authors are listed below in no particular or meaningful order other than separation into two sections, the first being science and the latter self-help. Many authors have produced several books; hence, the titles are omitted, but can readily be found on internet search engines. Countless other articles have been read to help me put together a coherent arc to the book and fill in educational gaps. I have greedily and unashamedly used the contents of this mass of literature without, I hope, stepping into plagiarism or copyright infringement. Please forgive me if this disclosure falls short of your desired acknowledgement. Also, in my attempt at humor I may have inadvertently stepped on some toes, but let me say that I have nothing but respect and admiration for all these authors, and any seeming belittlement just reflects my own brash clumsiness.

Science authors:

Thomas McFarlane, Louann Brizendine, Robert Wright, Max Tegmark, Victor Stenger, Amit Goswami, Johnjoe McFadden, Michael Shermer, David Deutsch, Ian Glynn, Evan Harris Walker, Tor Norretranders, Fred Alan Wolf, Isaac Asimov, Richard Feynman, Jagdish Mehra, Nigel Calder, Richard Morris, Roger Penrose, Richard Dawkins, Stephen Hawking, Leonard Mlodinow, Nick Herbert, Albert Einstein, Lisa Randall, Simon Singh, Carl Sagan, Ann Druyan, Michio Kaku, Bart Bok, Lawrence Jerome,

Virginia Postrel, David Halberstern, Julian Barbour, Stephen Gould, Ray Kurzweil, Milton and Rose Friedman, Thomas Sowell, Herman Kahn, Shintaro Ishihara, Cordelia Fine, the Dalai Lama, Howard Cutler, Deepak Chopra, Susan Greenfield, Steven Pinker, Aldous Huxley, James Christian, Sheila Ostrander, Lynn Shroeder, Alvin Toffler, Fritjof Capra, Erich Fromm, Sharon Begley, Desmond Morris, Greg DiJacobs, John Brockman, Jeffrey Schwartz, Robert Ornstein, Allan Hobson, Amir DiAczel, and Arthur Clarke.

Self-help authors:

Vernon Howard, Lucinda Bassett, Wayne Dyer, Robert Greene, Mark Hansen, Peter McWilliams, Tom Smith, Wendy Cooper, Scott Ventrella, Carol Adrienne, James Padfield, Terry Cole Whittaker, Marcus Allen , John Cleese, Robin Skynner, Philip Mcgraw, Leo Buscaglia, Lynn Grabhorne, Daniel Lapin, Larry Winget, Adrian Gostick, Chester Elton, Anthony Robbins, Eckhart Tolle, Ben Stein, Brian Tracey, Maxwell Maltz, Stephen Covey, Mihaly Csikzenmihali, Dennis Waitley, Roger Fisher, William Ury, Robert Shemin, Susan Jeffers, Paul Brunton, Norman Vincent Peale, Napoleon Hill, Ian McMahan, Dale Carnegie, Joseph Murphy, Ashley Montagu, Randolph Nesse, George Williams, Louise Hay, David Hilfiker, Louise Erdrich, Bernie Seigel, Norman Cousins, Harville Hendrix, Helen Hunt, Rhonda Byrne, Jack Canfield, and Laura Schlessinger.

And, of course, my publisher and editor.

Thank you all,

Lancaster Adams,

Orange County, California

INTRODUCTION

"The last thing in nature that man will understand
is the performance of his brain."
—John C. Eccles, 1977, scientist

You have read all the self-help books. It is the grand American obsession: improving yourself, pulling yourself up by your own bootstraps. Growth, change, and success are your goals. You repeat your affirmations of health, wealth, love, laughter, and success, regularly, endlessly, and persistently. But does it work? Are you just wasting your precious time? Is there any evidence or scientific support for all the New Age proclamations?

An occasional out of the blue check, chance meeting, opportunity, job offer, or phone call confirms your belief that it DOES work. But is it just random? Are you deluding yourself with wishful thinking? Can you really control your thoughts and project them "out there" to achieve your chosen goals? Does a creeping self-doubt at the edges of your mind tell you it's all just bogus, and to forget it?

Current experiments show that your brain utilizes about ten watts of electricity per second. That's enough juice to power a small flashlight. Thoughts of words and intended limb movements can be picked up from your brain with electrodes and read by computers. This information in turn can move cursors on computer screens.

So thoughts are real, tangible, concrete electrical events that can be detected outside your head. So perhaps your self-improvement gurus are on to something. This book helps you further explore some of the knowns and unknowns.

These neurological recorded events displayed on computer screens rely on conventionally understood electromagnetic transmissions. As such, they probably do not account for the purported quasi-magical magnetism, universal subconscious, or laws of attraction declared by many self-help authors.

It is in the poorly understood quantum realm that the concept of thought projection or resonance may be examined for the validity of the almost universal self-help proclamation of projecting our thoughts "out there." These "spooky effects at a distance," in Einstein's words, will be explored in light of current understanding and conjecture on the nature of consciousness in the human brain.

One personal account with a probable extrasensory perception (ESP) experience will be indulged in, together with some of the questions such experiences raise. Although this is anecdotal and does not reach the criteria of statistical exactitude expected by you the reader, it does serve as an example by which to explore together the fascinating phenomena which inspire and enthrall both self-help writers and readers alike.

> *"No pleasure is comparable to the study upon the*
> *vantage ground of truth."*
> —Francis Bacon

CONTENTS

CHAPTER ONE

ELECTRICITY AND THE HUMAN BRAIN

*"Electricity is actually made up of extremely tiny particles
called electrons, that you cannot see with the naked eye unless you
have been drinking."*
—Dave Barry, humorist

Our brain's cerebral cortex contains up to thirty-three billion neurons, each with ten thousand synaptic connections. The electrical pulses along the wires or axons to these electrical junctions or synapses represent the bulk of our brain's electrical output. There are about 62,000 miles of axons (those insulated or myelinated nerve fibers) in each of our heads. The total energy consumption of our brain is twenty-five watts per second. About ten watts of this is used in computation. This neuronal mass with all its computations, believed to be similar to algorithms processed in a neural net computer, is thought to constitute our unconscious or subconscious mind. This is about ninety-nine point nine percent of our brain's activity which runs on automatic.

Remarkably, this electricity in the brain can be detected, fed into a computer, and used to initiate the movement of a cursor on a computer screen. These experiments entailed patients whose skulls had been partially removed for other brain surgery, and the electrical signals were detected from electrodes placed directly on the brain tissue, in this initial work. Thick bone weakened the signal strength, hampering electrical signal detection.

Incredibly, movement-generating thoughts create electrical brain waves that can now be detected and decoded outside our human brains. Notwithstanding the challenge posed by the human cranium, electrodes placed outside the skull can also detect electrical brainwaves. With a skullcap of electrodes recording their thoughts, some patients exhibited the ability to pick out letters on a computer. Even monkeys' thoughts can be detected outside their brains, then deciphered and used to send signals to an artificial hand to play notes on a piano.

Detecting thoughts from human minds is now so commonplace that ordinary people can actually buy headsets that can read their own thoughts for less than a hundred dollars. The brainwaves picked up whilst watching a movie can be sent to a computer, which will then change the ending of the movie (for example, to save the heroine) just by using the willed thoughts of the movie watcher. Thoughts really are actual things.

This shows conclusively, without any shadow of doubt, several key facts. Thoughts are real, not some nebulous gossamer to be philosophized about. Some physicists go so far as to say that philosophy is dead, as it is all conjecture without facts. Scientific experiments provide facts that can be used to prove or disprove assertions. Thoughts are not some imagined parapsychological, noetic mumbo jumbo. They have electrical properties. They can be detected outside the head. They can be read by computers. These thoughts can range from thoughts of movement to directed selection of letters.

Miraculously, we can develop software that amplifies these signals, and actually understands the human sender's intent and purpose. Weak and jumbled with all the other electrical noise our brains produce, conscious thought, which we are aware of and create, together with the choices being made by acts of will, can be detected outside our heads.

A common thread found in most self-help books is the exposition that our thoughts travel out beyond our bodies into the environment, and impact events. Be that as it may, they are correct in characterizing thoughts as real, tangible concrete things, and yes, they do escape the physical confines of our brains when conditions are right.

Other parts of the electromagnetic spectrum, those with weak fields of electromagnetism, are generated by the mass of neurons which conduct the activity of our subconscious. These force fields become ordered into synchronous brain waves that are less than 0.1% of our total mental output. Some believe that these synchronous brain waves are the substance of our consciousness.

Much work has been done studying the brain states of experienced meditators. It appears that meditation can improve the generation of synchronous brain waves, such as alpha waves. This may account for the altered state of consciousness that experienced meditators claim they achieve, with increased awareness and insight.

Prior to experimental physics, this kind of deep thought, sometimes aided by ecstasy-type drugs, was considered the mainstay of mankind's search for the truth, and the vehicle for exploration of the boundaries of human knowledge. Lacking experimental verification, it was the purview of the philosophical and religious elite. Scientific results are now broadcast daily to the wider public through the electronic media and, if repeatable, become readily accepted by the masses and incorporated into their worldview.

Results from the labs of the neuroscientists show that the physics of brain signals is clear. The electromagnetic outputs emanating from our brains are real. However, they are extremely weak, with much noise, and decline rapidly in strength as one moves inches away from the skull. The signals require much amplification, filtering, and organization in order to be picked up more than a hand-width from your body. This complicates the self-help-book claims that they embody enough power to project your thoughts, including affirmations and visualizations, "out there" into the universe.

Nevertheless, with respect to informational content, these signals do indeed seem to meet the requirements necessary to be consistent with the self-help book's advice on the focus of one's thoughts. Commanding one's thoughts appears to be an imperative for self-improvement, regardless of the actual mechanism. What you do with those thoughts then redirects your life.

"If you want to be happy, set a goal that commands your thoughts, liberates your energy, and inspires your hopes"
—Andrew Carnegie, industrialist and philanthropist

CHAPTER TWO

RECEPTION OF ELECTROMAGNETISM
BY THE HUMAN BRAIN

"Purple Haze all in my brain,
Lately things don't seem the same,
Actin' funny, but I don't know why,
'Scuse me while I kiss the sky."
—Jimi Hendrix, *Purple Haze*, 1967

What about reception? Can the human brain receive electromagnetic signals from outside our heads? Will the signal and reception be subtle enough to provide the human with useful information, or just a sledgehammer burst of energy that disorients him, like Jimi Hendrix's purple haze?

Magnetism, artificially applied in the form of transcranial magnetic stimulation (TMS), does disengage brain areas for fractions of a second. This indicates that yes, magnetic fields outside the head can impact our brain, and ultimately our thoughts.

Even as early as 1866, in the treatise *Medical Common Sense*, the brain was understood to be receptive to electricity, although its vagueness reflected the state of then-current knowledge: "The brain is the great receiving and distributing reservoir of vital electricity, just as the heart is the receiving and distributing reservoir of blood."

Will our state of knowledge fifty years hence enable us to

definitively change thoughts using distant electromagnetic waves? Well, it's not for lack of trying, as both the Russian and American defense departments have been experimenting with this for decades. Much of this work remains classified. Although weapons-grade high energy pulses can disable or disorient men subjected to these powerful insults to the delicate neurochemistry of their brains, whether or not actual thoughts can be transmitted or changed at lower energy levels is not revealed.

What is known in the TMS work is that in order to shut down the brain for short bursts of time, the TMS magnetic coil is placed in close proximity to the skull. The transmission of magnetic signals over greater distances would require much larger transmitters, certainly beyond the power of the three-pound lump of grey matter that is our human brain's generating capacity. Unless some amplification system exists in the universe outside our heads, then the self-help books' claims of receiving input from the "universe," "universal mind or subconscious," or inter-human transmission initiated via electromagnetism generated within someone else's head, appears to be severely challenged.

"It may well be that there is something else going on in the brain that we don't have an inkling of at the moment."
—Roger Penrose, mathematician, scientist

Out-of-body experiences have been reported by both trauma victims near death, and experienced meditators. These have been called paranormal, but the more science uncovers about the brain the more we find what was once paranormal becomes subsumed into normal, natural biology.

Magnetic pulses applied externally along the sides of the head overlying the temporal lobes of the cerebral cortex, specifically a region called the right angular gyrus, produce these weird out-of-body experiences, particularly the strange sensation of floating two feet above one's own body, looking down on it. This has been made popular in TV documentaries sensationally claiming paranormal near death experiences, but in this case, it is just a malfunction of the brain's receiving external magnetic energy.

Statistics bore both layman and scientist alike. Simply put, mankind did not evolve to think statistically. Indeed, there are remote tribes in Borneo who cannot comprehend or use numbers above the count of three. Proving the existence to hard-headed scientists of self-help books' claims of reception directly by the human brain, without bothering with the usual channels of television, book, or telephone, relies heavily on statistics.

Most folks understand that tossing a coin one hundred times will get them about fifty heads and fifty tails. This is the normal result of chance. If the result varies greatly from 50:50 then something is afoot and needs investigation. For instance, the coin may be weighted more on one side than the other, thus disturbing its balance, and giving say, seventy heads and thirty tails after a hundred tosses. At any rate, *something* is influencing the outcome of the toss. It is a reality. It is a fact, particularly if the hundred-toss game is repeated many times with different observers, yet still garnering the 70:30 result.

If two people are sitting in different, unconnected, soundproofed, windowless rooms, and one of them turns a card marked with, say, a circle, or a cross, or other simple geometric form on it, and the person in the other room can guess it correctly seventy out of a hundred times, then statistically this is significant, reflecting a reality. This, if reproducible many times, is factually relevant. What is going on?

As it happens, there are some special individuals who have the power to do this reproducibly. Cheating in the form of surreptitious communication between the two people was ruled out by using stringent university-based studies. The conclusion drawn was that some people do indeed have real paranormal powers. Other researchers have contested the results, but cannot completely rule them out either.

This opens a window into the abilities of some human brains to "see" at a distance, known as remote viewing, without the use of the five senses of sight, sound, touch, taste and smell. This is called extrasensory perception, or ESP.

Russian and American scientists, in different experiments, have enclosed some of these gifted individuals in devices known as Faraday cages, which shield the enclosed person from electrical and radio signals, but not from extremely low frequencies or light. These seers were still able to achieve statistically significant ESP "hits," or correct calls of picture cards turned in an enclosed room at some distance from them. This would indicate information transfer occurred without the participation of the normal electromagnetic spectrum. Interestingly, electrical activity of our human brains is thought to create its own Faraday cage effect, which evolved to protect us from the ever-present electromagnetic activity sweeping our earthly home.

> *"No indeed; I don't know anything. You see I'm stuffed,*
> *so I have no brains at all."*
> —The Scarecrow, *The Wonderful Wizard of Oz*

Notwithstanding this fascinating scenario that ESP is a real phenomenon, with information both coming *and* going, transfer *and* reception by gifted individuals using currently unknown channels outside the electromagnetic spectrum, skepticism (Do you take us for scarecrows?!) rightly abounds. In 1988 the US National Research Council reviewed one hundred and thirty years of this ESP research and concluded that the statistics were not valid. The slight rates of positive hits above normal chance were not believed to be statistically significant enough, nor reproducible in normal folks.

So, what if anything can be concluded from these contradictory assessments? What is the truth? In science one individual report is anecdotal, and results must be repeatedly reproduced to be accepted as factual truth. Yet some special individuals did score much higher than chance at guessing cards. Faraday cages, included the inbuilt one created by our own brain's electrical activity, did not block their gifts. Transfer of information occurred through some medium or back channel outside the electromagnetic spectrum, but the question is, how? Perhaps our fundamental mechanistic understanding of reality has no path or energy that our machines would detect for these phenomena.

Obsessive-compulsive disorder leads to actions such as compulsive repetitive hand washing, constantly checking that you have turned out the lights, and even returning home over and over, just to recheck that you set the locks. When drugs and behavioral training fail, applying electrical pulses to the brain reduces this activity, along with depression and anxiety, by fifty percent. Our brains do pick up and respond to external electromagnetism, without recourse to witchcraft or other paranormal interventions.

Your self-help literature is insistent that your thoughts, when sufficiently focused, are projected out beyond yourself, somehow resonating with the stuff of the universe, which then feeds back required information to achieve your goals. Being "open for reception" is an oft-repeated mantra. What evidence is there that life can perceive signals outside the familiar five senses?

The earth's natural electromagnetic field and the sun's solar waves have been with us throughout evolution in various forms to which our brains have had to adapt. One field that surrounds the earth is derived from its iron core, which being liquid sloshes around beneath our feet. Migratory birds have evolved mechanisms to detect this magnetic field and use it as their own personal GPS system for navigation.

Humans too can pick up magnetic fields, and react to them. This is not considered a "sense," in that unless they are unusually and unnaturally strong, we don't perceive or become aware of them, but they can and do alter our brains. Alternating magnetic fields outside our skulls are received by our brains. They begin to dance in tune with them. Our brains mimic or follow the pulsing they create, disrupting normal brain wave patterns. As some consider our brain waves to be eliciting our consciousness, this could be of some consequence, if exposure was continual. In primates, exposure to alternating magnetic fields can induce immediate physical violence. Birds can lose their sense of direction. Cancers can be created. Recent studies with humans show that magnetic stimulation of the appropriate brain areas induced right-handed people to become left-handed and use their left hands as their primary dominant hand.

Patents have been filed for remotely monitoring and altering brain waves using these technologies coupled with directional antennas as early as 1976. Whether or not these patent technologies have been developed and exploited is unknown. However, various defense agencies have held closely guarded secret research projects on human reception of various electromagnetic signals to induce behavioral changes in recipients, unknowing or otherwise.

Disorientation is common with powerful enough blasts, which is unsurprising to those of us who nuke our pizza in the microwave oven for supper.

But again, there is probably a lot more going on that we cannot yet conceptualize. As a young boy growing up in England I readily devoured all that my biology, chemistry, and physics teachers fed me. As my intellect slowly awakened, the first original thought I recall, around age fourteen, was: perhaps our brains have not evolved for us to EVER to be able to understand how all this works. Of course this was not an original thought to the rest of mankind, and had been mooted much earlier by a far greater intellect than mine:

> *"The Universe is not only queerer than we suppose,*
> *but queerer than we can suppose."*
> —Haldane, 1927, biologist

CHAPTER THREE

QUESTIONS OF QUANTUM CONSCIOUSNESS

"In my Father's house are many mansions."
—Jesus Christ, John 14:2

This, of course, is open to many interpretations; however, the multiple universe theory leaps readily to mind, although its link to quantum events inside our heads is a long and intellectually challenging road. With such a delicious topic as quantum consciousness, the lead-in to this chapter warrants not one, but two quotations:

"There are more things in heaven and earth, Horatio, than are dreamt of in your philosophy."
—William Shakespeare, *Hamlet,* 1601

How our consciousness arises in our brain is not yet known, and may not be knowable.

This opens the door for snake-oil salesmen, but also still represents one of the finest venues for scientific exploration by our striving intellects. Our evolution has patched together our brains from whatever spare parts were available on that long, long road from our primeval ancestors. Brains were not designed, and their primary functions were food, survival and sex.

Philosophers have struggled through the ages, using their considerable intellectual prowess to think deeply through mechanisms that may create our different levels of consciousness. No consensus has been found, although the synchronous force fields generated from the electromagnetic force field of the mass of the brain's neurons is gaining traction. Although it is possibly easier to visualize these waves billowing or hovering *above* the brain, in all probability they involve the very matter of the brain itself, continually flooding or immersing different parts of the brain with their synchronous pulsing.

Scientists work with facts, experimentation, and reproducible results to parse out the different mental modalities from which consciousness emerges. No one knows how. Perhaps it is beyond our ken to understand, requiring new dimensions and better models of physics. Nevertheless, the yearning, the desire to know more than our banal, mundane, humdrum existence, reverberates through most races and societies. In the past, religions filled this role. Today, Americans' current obsession with self-help affirmations reflects a religious undertone. This is particularly emphasized when coupled with the belief in the power of one's thoughts to project out into the universe and change circumstances and future events.

In the past, psychologists have labeled this wishful thinking in children "magical thinking." Children with their developing imaginations sometimes delude themselves that they cause events outside themselves, such as the rain or a parent's divorce, through what they have been thinking about. Scary, yet powerful at the same time. When adults practice it as a result of reading their self-help books, is it a similar delusion, or is there just a smidgen of reality underlying it, perhaps in the quantum world, awaiting the revelation of biophysics to give it a clear underpinning?

What is quantum physics? What is quantum consciousness? The great physicist Richard Feynman once declared that if someone told him that they understood quantum physics, then he knew that they *didn't* understand quantum physics! Quantum physics replaces our understanding of the normal Newtonian mechanics of our big, seeable, touchable world, as we approach the size of the atom. Then everything gets really weird.

Imagine you went to a farm, looked into a field and saw a cow, but the cow could be in two different parts of the field *at the same time*, until you chose to watch it munch grass in your corner. Your very act of gaping at it fixes it where you first observe it.

Impossible and crazy, you might say in our large-object world, but this is what the physicists tell us happens all the time with subatomic particles.

Matter does not just devolve to smaller and smaller particles. At the submicroscopic level matter vacillates between tiny particles and waves, then ultimately just energy.

These subatomic particles can seemingly be present in two locations at the same time, or jump between positions. This quantum activity can change the way the parent molecule behaves depending on which position the subatomic particle fixes itself. What is truly weird is that the act of human observation somehow acts to fix the position of the jumpy wavelike particle. Thankfully for our sanity, as molecular size increases, this quantum activity appears to get swamped by the density and noise of all the concurrent quantum activity, something physicists call decoherence, and when we see a cow in a field all alone on its lonesome, it really, really *is* just one cow.

The flux of electrical activity in the sixty-two thousand miles of neurons and neurochemical interchange across billions of synapse connections is thought to create quantum energy fields that ebb back and forth across and within our brains in never-ending dances, and constitute our consciousness. Of course this is still conjecture, and no one can categorically to state it as fact, leaving room for a little hocus-pocus and exploitive charlatans, but most self-help book authors do not fall into that category. They appear to be firmly convinced believers in their creed.

Can science bolster these believers? Imaging our brains as we think thoughts can monitor activity that is associated with thought. Technology such as the PET scanner (positron emitter topography) identifies metabolic activity in patches of the brain, after pre-loading the body with radioactive tracers, indicating areas of the brain being used for these thinking tasks. Tracking sensations and emotions as they occur can be observed with fMRI (functional Magnetic Resonance Imaging), showing which parts of the brain are handling these tasks in real time. What emerges from these studies is the concept of the conscious mind as a constantly fluctuating mosaic of force fields over different areas of our brains as we think thoughts. But this is still geography; sophisticated, yes, but basically mapping out brain regions associated with different jobs.

"The human brain, then, is the most complicated organization of matter that we know."
—Isaac Asimov, prolific science fiction author

In states of deep meditation the Buddhist Dalai Lama, who is well-read in quantum physics, states that he can "see" events on the other side of the universe in real time.

Einstein showed us that, in our universe at least, there is a speed limit on the electromagnetic spectrum, the speed of light, a little under seven hundred million miles per hour, which is a bit more than my Dad's old Ford van could manage downhill, but a speed limit nevertheless. Thus, the speed at which information can be transferred using electromagnetic waves is policed by Einstein's speed limit. Your self-help books' conviction of human brain broadcasting and reception would have to submit to this cosmic law, if electromagnetism is the medium of transfer.

But wait: quantum physics permits the *instantaneous* transfer of information, albeit on a teeny-weeny scale, across distances, without regard to the seven hundred million miles-per-hour speed limit set by our traffic cop Einstein. So, put away your radar gun and ticket book, and let us try and understand. Experiments with subatomic particles clearly and repeatedly show that the act of observing one bit of matter that had been in contact, or "entangled," with a second bit of matter affects the orientation of this second bit of matter *instantaneously*.

Even more fascinating is the fact that these two subatomic flecks of matter can interact instantaneously with each other even if they are *miles and miles apart*. Weird doesn't even come close to describing this crazy quantum world. What is even more devastating to our treasured sense of order and logic in our universe is the additional fact that it is the intervention of human thought, that of the experimenter, to choose the timing of the measurement of the first particle's orientation which determines when and how the second particle reacts. Amazing stuff indeed.

How can that be? Even Einstein was shook up about it, deriding this entangled effect of separated particles as "spooky effects at a distance." Scientists and doctors may confuse the lay person with the arcane terminology they use for mental short-cuts and attempts at exactitude, and are often accused of attempting to baffle us with "baloney sandwiches." Physicists describe the activities described in the cow analogy thus: superposition is the seeming ability of a subatomic particle to be two places at once; non-locality is Einstein's spooky effects at a distance; and collapse of the wave function potential is the act of choosing to observe the subatomic particle, thus fixing it in reality.

How can this be? How can something be in two places at once? How can a particle change the state of another particle miles away? How do Einstein's spooky effects at a distance work? How can thinking and choosing to observe one speckle of matter affect something across the horizon? It would be nice to know and understand in depth, but for the purpose of this book, acceptance will work and bring us closer to possible explanations for the claims of your self-help literature. The great inventor Thomas Alva Edison was reputedly cornered by a persistent woman at a dinner party, demanding an explanation of how his electricity worked. After several unsuccessful attempts, Edison just exploded and said, "It is electricity, Madam, just use it!"

Oliver Wendell Holmes, the Supreme Court justice, exhorted us to "think things, not words….catchwords can delay further analysis for fifty years!" So who knows, and who can know? It just is, and it's true, a real, hard, inconvenient fact.

Another fact, which relies more on mathematical physics than direct experimental observation (as CNN wasn't there to record it) is that once upon a time, at the singularity of the Big Bang from which our universe expanded, *ALL* bits of matter were "entangled."

Thus all bits of matter, or subatomic particles, as the elements had not had time to form yet, were in intimate contact with each other, or entangled. Their chemical descendents now make up us humans. That also applies to our brains. All the subatomic particles that form our brain matter were once squished together in an incredibly dense lump, undergoing who knows what kind of intercourse and comingling. Victorian propriety would have been shocked.

Can exploration of the rare reported ESP events recursively open a window into the quantum mechanics of consciousness for the physicists to investigate? Currently they are bogged down in string theory, ten-plus dimensions, dark matter and energy, disputes over the very existence of time and gravity, and multiple universes, but it's all in their heads with precious little experimentation to back it up. Challenges abound, but that's what humans rise to.

One problem is that of scale. How can two tiny, separated but entangled bits of matter or energy impact something as large as the real-time processing of a thought?

Amplification or leverage is needed.

"Give me a lever long enough and a fulcrum on which to place it and I shall move the world."
—Archimedes, Greek philosopher, 250 BC

Thought itself is measurable as an electrical discharge using electroencephalographic electrodes on your head. Thought, however, is a much, much bigger event than one casually altered spin of one of a pair of subatomic particles. Where is the amplification or leverage if quantum events are responsible for the instantaneous transformation to and from human brains? This massive difference in scale is important in understanding this process, if indeed it occurs, because the math and physics change as we approach real, life-sized measurable activity.

Your self-help books require belief in the ability of humans to project and receive thoughts. Anecdotes abound, but the science is lacking. How is it possible, or is it even possible, that a focused thought can be projected out into the universe? Even more beguiling is the question of how such a thought be instantaneously perceived by another sentient being.

Answers are elusive, but will be attempted later on in this book and quantum events will be the starting point. What, if any proof is there of quantum consciousness? Debates rage in books devoted to this topic, but one sure thing emerges: quantum events do occur within the human brain.

The brain is composed of molecules whose intrinsic particles undergo the whirl of quantum activity just as every other molecule on the planet that is above the inertia level of absolute zero temperature, which even then may be permitted. Your computers and calculators operate through quantum mechanics, with subatomic particles appearing instantaneously in different locations within their chips and undergoing energy jumps in a skittish directed dance. Can such jumps alter the function of our brain's neurons, and thus our very thoughts? Some scientists believe it so.

"It was about three o'clock at night when the final result of the calculation [which gave birth to quantum mechanics] lay before me. At first I was deeply shaken. I was so excited that I could not think of sleep. So I left the house and awaited the sunrise on a rock."
—Werner Heisenberg, discoverer of the Uncertainty Principle

So shaken was Heisenberg, he had to resort to humor about what his work had uncovered, with all its earth-shattering implications for mankind.

"There are things that are so serious,
that you can only joke about them."
—Werner Heisenberg, quantum physicist

CHAPTER FOUR

LIGHTS IN THE ATTIC?

*"Light and matter are both single entities and the apparent duality
arises from the limitations of our language"*
—Werner Heisenberg, quantum physicist

In 2010, Chinese scientists reported their ability to change two entangled photons, separated by a distance of ten miles of open space, solely by changing the initial photon in their lab. This repeats with photons the earlier work reported elsewhere on altering the spin of subatomic particles at a distance, or non-locality. The press labeled the Chinese work "teleportation," or the transfer of information across a distance without use of conventional electro-magnetic means.

Many of you reading this may remember your high school biology teacher explaining photosynthesis to you. Without this capture and conversion of the sun's energy, life on earth, including us humans, would not exist. It's that important. Photosynthesis is now known to result from the capture of a packet of light energy, or photon, by the plant's chlorophyll in a quantum manner. The photon is absorbed in various ways depending on the most energy efficient pathway extant in the plant at the time, and ultimately yields its energy by displacing an electron, causing it to jump to a higher energy level. This changed molecule can then trigger a series of chemical steps that produces sugar as a storage medium. This is quantum mechanics at work in biology.

"And God said, let there be light: and there was light. "
—Genesis 1:3

Incongruously, the converse is thought to happen within your head. Your skin has a pigment, melanin, to absorb UV energy to help protect you from the sun's rays. This pigment is also found within the pitch-black darkness of your brain. What is it doing there where the sun don't shine? Is there a reason we keep our brains in the dark?

Do we just have to rely on the biblical separation of darkness from light as the way it is, or is something else happening in those gloomy recesses?

*"And God saw the light, that it was good: and God divided the light
from the darkness."*
—Genesis 1:4

Although melanin is distributed unevenly throughout our brains, one place it usually concentrates is the substantia nigra. In patients suffering from Parkinson's disease, whose brains show a deficit of the essential neurotransmitter dopamine, their substantia nigra areas show a loss of melanin. Interestingly, the neurotransmitters dopamine, adrenaline, and noradrenaline are made in chemical steps from the amino acid tyrosine, which is also a building block of melanin. The fact that melanin shares a common pathway of production in the brain has led some to consider melanin as a potential source, or reservoir, for neurotransmitter production. Could quantum nudges to our brain's melanin spawn the release of neurotransmitters? Could these quantum events be initiated elsewhere outside our heads? Neurotransmitter release would certainly alter our thoughts.

Melanin, or in the brain neuromelanin, which comes in various shades from yellow through brown, is known to absorb photons. The Chinese work shows that photons can hop across space instantaneously and transfer information at the same time. Can the melanin in our heads be affected thus? Do photons teleport between our brains?

For those of you unfortunate enough to have landed up in your hospital emergency room with an allergic reaction or a hornet sting, you will remember the agony of laryngospasm, as your windpipe swelled up and your breathing became tenuous just before you passed out for lack of oxygen. Your doctor probably ordered you a shot of adrenaline. As this has happened to me, let me assure you that the adrenaline surge that sweeps through your body creates an instant rush of well-being and feels very enjoyable, considering what went before. Imagine, then, the effect of little squirts of adrenaline between the synapses of your brain, and how that could alter your mentation.

Should melanin be involved in adrenaline production in your brain, and that in turn results from the quantum reception of photons (either internal, or external as in our self-help model), then amplification or leverage is readily seen. Flooding synapses with neurochemicals derived from the single quantum interaction photon or other subatomic particle with melanin would create a cascade of neurochemical events that could eventually lead to new thoughts.

Other possible roles for melanin exist, both in isolation or in combination with the above conjectures. Could your brain melanin be there just as a sponge to soak up or accept photons released as by products in your brain, or spurious non-signaling photons bombarding your head from the external environment? Melanin, in itself a semiconductor with switching capabilities, is also able to absorb free radicals in addition to photons. One role may be to accept photons from quantum events in your brain. As electrons jump in quantum fashion from one energy level to another, photons can be released, and the melanin could act as a buffer to absorb them and protect the brain from short circuits.

If photons can pop into our heads from the outside, a question posed by the Chinese teleportation experiments, they also may interact with neurons and create an electrical, and not necessarily a neurochemical, response. Some neurons are always to be found within the brain that are ready to fire.

The pores or channels on their axons, which permit the influx of sodium ions in which they are bathed and thus trigger nerve firing, have a molecular lid on them which can be open or closed. This mechanism is sensitive to the molecular configuration of the proteins of which the lid is made. This configuration can be modified by very small quantum differences, or superpositions of protons, similar to a light touch on a mousetrap snapping it shut. The energy of the photon can be sufficient to bring about this change, thus ultimately firing the nerve, then its compatriots, in a cascading multiplier, leveraged amplification process. Thoughts can then begin.

Thinking of photons as just quanta of light tends to mask our thinking; as Heisenberg suggested, they are also packets of energy capable of transmitting information. Our language, reflecting eons of evolution, is still inadequate when it comes to describing the behavior of our subatomic world.

Both chemical and electrical events, and probably both in combination, can be leveraged out of single-photon entanglement with the existing structures in melanin and nerve fiber pores. Photons are not necessarily lights in the attics of our heads, but potential emissaries, initiators, and promulgators of our thoughts. Exciting though this may be, little proof has been experimentally achieved. The questions and conjectures raised in this chapter can only be addressed with more research, which is why God created graduate students and research grants.

CHAPTER FIVE

IS THIS ESP?

"True I talk of Dreams,
Which are the children of an idle brain,
Begot of nothing but vain fantasy"
—Shakespeare, *Romeo and Juliet*

Are there other avenues to explore quantum consciousness? Do some of our dreams provide a glimpse of quantum transfer between people? Can the strictures of modern research ever be applied to a common, but nebulous, human occurrence? Is it all the gibberish of vain fantasy, as proclaimed by Shakespeare? Or worse, is it the mental disturbance of sleep deprivation, as proclaimed by England's latter-day poets?

"You know I can't sleep, I can't stop my brain"
—The Beatles, *I'm So Tired*

Current sleep researchers believe their work indicates that the rapid eye movement (REM) stage of sleep is when dreams occur. This was discovered by rudely waking up poor volunteers in sleep labs, just when they were settling into a nice juicy dream.

Furthermore, most dreams are now thought, through experiments such as these, to be a recollection, filtering, and filing of your day's events, and integrating them with your long-term memories through interaction with the histones attached to the DNA in the lower temporal lobes of your long-term memory bank. Your short-term memory is believed to be housed in your hippocampus, which is then downloaded during dreams and incorporated into the memories that make you unique. This is why napping aids students swotting for exams. Short-term memory of data is shunted into areas for long-term recall during their naps.

Interestingly, physically fit kids do better on memory tests than slackers, and also have a twelve percent larger hippocampus than the goof-offs. Some other unique individuals have been studied and found to have enlargement of these brain memory areas. Fortunately, or unfortunately, these patients have the incredible ability to recall from memory everything that has happened during their lives day by day, hour by hour, in a chronologically correct and verifiable fashion. Not what you might wish, but there you have it. We still have much to learn about what some of our brains are capable of in special people.

Can other types of dreams exist, outside the mundane chore of shuttling memories out of our hippocampus? Do some rare dreams permit communication across great distances? Would they qualify as being fed by quantum non-local input from outside our heads? You may be helped in reaching your decision to the answers to these vexing questions, if you will permit the self-indulgence of the author to relate one anecdotal dream that contained factual, timely, actionable, information from far across the sea.

By way of background, my father was a stoic Lancastrian, never given to complaining of aches or pains and always ready with a laugh or two. Parsimonious, or cheap, as my spouse accused the family, this frugality extended to the use (or lack thereof) of phone calls in the day when transatlantic telephone calls were more expensive than they are today. Communications between California and Liverpool were therefore restricted to infrequent handwritten letters and Christmas cards.

Dream scientists tell us that the dreams that unfold during our REM sleep, discarding the junk, can be soundless, still snapshots, movies, black and white, or in color.

Dreams are normal for everyone, and do not reflect hallucination, psychosis, or schizophrenia. Most of us forget our dreams when we wake up and get on with our day, and even if prodded by annoying sleep lab scientists for recall on awakening, only remember snapshots of jumbled incoherent thoughts. This is why we are programmed to forget most of our dreams instantly, as the information is garbled with the junk.

Back to our story; after a two- or three-month spell of no letters or calls that would prime, prompt, cue, or fuel dreams of the green, green grass of home, I went to bed at my usual time after an uneventful day. I then dreamt a dream that has transformed my life.

My father appeared to me in my dream in a most unusual position. There was no sound. There was no auditory hallucination one associates with schizophrenia to accompany this vivid series of moving, colored images. The dream was sharp, clear, strong, and repetitive. The unmistakable image of my father was insistent, with a pronounced configuration of his posture. He repeatedly turned his broad back to me, something he had never done while I was growing up with him. In addition, whilst in this position he repeatedly placed his arm behind his back, itself an abnormal anatomical posture, and pointed with his finger to the middle of his spine. This was repeated in seemingly real time four or five times, lasting what felt like five minutes. It was persistent, very powerfully felt, and unyielding. My dad was showing me his back and pointing to it over and over again.

On awakening, I vividly recalled the dream. I mentioned it to my spouse and did something very unusual for me with my frugal north country upbringing: I called home from California to Liverpool. My mother answered the phone, and after the customary short preliminaries, I asked how dad was. Her answer floored me.

"Oh luv, its funny you called; he hurt his back digging the garden and they've just taken him to the hospital for tests."

Dumbfounded, I told Mum of my dream and the reason I had called. She took it in her stride, being an old North Country woman, who always taught us kids that truth was stranger than fiction, and "there's nowt so queer as folk," then gave me the hospital phone number. She had never herself evinced any so-called psychic abilities during the war or our growing up, but we both knew that Dad had in the past.

I called Dad's hospital. As I am a medical doctor with a stint in cancer research, and still retain my English accent, I was able to cajole, bully, and plead my way through the arcane English NHS system to get to speak to him. Yes, he said, he was in intense pain in the middle of his back. No, he had no recollection of any dream with me, and in his usual blunt manner, told me not to be soft in the head like a Yank.

He was proud that his son was now a doctor, and eagerly relayed his symptoms and asked my advice. The X-rays had come back showing a lesion at the T-5 level of his spine in the middle of his back. Dad had cut back from his forty Woodbine cigarettes a day habit under my urging, but that had been too late to prevent the previously unknown carcinoma growing in his lungs, then metastasizing to his spine. He died after it spread to his brain in about six months, after some very shabby treatment in the English socialized medicine system.

My father was a remarkable man in many ways, a decorated war hero after storming the Normandy beaches with the other lads and fighting his way across the Third Reich up to the Kiel canal near the Russian front. However, what is relevant to this chapter on the possibility of ESP through dreams is the unequivocal evidence of a dream that Dad underwent and relayed to us when we were children.

After the war, England was impoverished and under the gloomy gray mantle of the new socialism; few families could afford to own a telephone. Communications were through visits among family every few weeks. Dad's dream was revealed to us children when he came down for breakfast. He was unusually disheveled for such a proud man, pale and drawn.

"My brother Walter's dead, I've been fighting with him all night," were the first words out of his lips, stunning us children. Our mother confirmed Dad's unusual restless sleep, telling us that he had been tossing and turning in their bed all night. Later that day, we had a visitor that brought the grim news. Dad's elder brother, Walter, had died unexpectedly in his sleep that same night.

Some coincidence, you may say. Death was not expected. No unusual illness was present, nor discussions made in the preceding weeks of any impending doom. The brothers loved each other, were on good speaking terms, and had no fraternal conflicts.

Yet, there is the dream, with its confirmation and its highly irregular struggle and prolonged content. The conclusion was absolute in Dad's mind when he spoke so forthrightly to us, his children. This was totally out of character, for him to relate something so highly personal as a dream. Dad kept his thoughts and feelings to himself.

My subsequent training as a scientist and doctor has not given me any way of explaining this strange dream and dramatic outcome. Dad's participatory dream predicted a real event, which we witnessed as fact, with our dead uncle. Dad's brain had picked up knowledge in an unconventional and physically expressed manner that turned out to be true.

He never ever got lucky with the football pools, though, more's the pity. This was not directed or willed percipient dreaming. It just happened to him. It was an extremely rare event in his life. It was not reproducible. It had intense, meaningful, emotional content. This "gift" was unsought and unasked for. This happened to a hard-boiled survivor who, though capable of deep love, was not given to belief in God, religion, or any fanciful creed, dismissing it all as "softness."

Returning to my own dream which I intimately experienced and for which I can vouchsafe, can it be construed as ESP? Or was I just soft in the head, as my Dad proclaimed? Did my father unknowingly and unwittingly, in his dire hour of need, communicate to his son the doctor, his pain and suffering that he would be hard put to share through his stoicism in a face-to-face conversation? Did my father's brain have some unusual chip that permitted both reception and transmission, on different occasions, of information across distance? It would appear something remarkable occurred in his head with his dream of his brother's death. But, this was different from what happened in my dream, as he had absolutely no recollection of any sort.

In my dream the facts are clear. The distance between father and son was six thousand miles. There was no sound. The dream played out over several minutes. The content was relevant, vivid, powerful, repetitive, persistent, insistent, and factually correct. That's a lot of stuff. It created action on my part. I was able to counsel, educate, and ameliorate suffering in another human being; small recompense for him, and those like him, who had stood alone during our island's darkest hour, then survived to usher in my generation.

My dream was not some mild, whimsical, or possibly hallucinatory vision. It was powerful and unrelenting. It was vivid. It forced me to take action. The image of my father pointing repeatedly at his midback, insisting I pay him attention, knowing that I was with him and watching him, were feelings irrevocably branded into my consciousness. How did this work? What were the signals?

This was a one-off event for me, with no priors and no similar call to action dreams since then. The out of the norm action for me back then was the transatlantic phone call. It was triggered by the intensity, duration, and highly relevant data dump of practical information contained in those mental images that flashed through my head. I do not consider myself psychic then or now, whatever that means. My stock market portfolio is stark testimony to my lame abilities at future predictions.

The key issue of this possible ESP event is the amount of information transferred, coupled with its assembly of moving usable and intelligible images in my mind's eye.

Quantum physicists tell us that too much information swamps quantum events with so much noise that signal strength is diluted to insignificance, or in their parlance, undergoes decoherence. Before we dismiss this ESP-type dream as failing to qualify as quantum dependent, it must be remembered that amplification steps can occur in our brains starting with simple quantum events as discussed earlier, and will be revisited in later chapters. This neither proves nor disproves quantum consciousness.

Any model that neurophysicists hammer together must encompass events such as these, unless they can develop alternate explanations as to what was going on. The onus is on the scientists, not those who experience these strange events, to develop a model that accounts for large amounts of data transmission and its subsequent reassembly into meaningful mental images. It will not be easy. Both quantum and electromagnetic transmission may have been involved, as there was a broad time window between the dream and the phone call. New physics may be needed, but this certainly represents a bona fide window on the mind. Unfortunately, one-off events are obviously not reproducible, a requirement for experimentation, and thus new theoretical postulates take priority.

As we leave this chapter on individual and highly personal esoterica, we can return to mechanisms that make your self-help books work. Self-discipline is available to everyone all the time, as it has been down through the ages. And it works.

For all of you who wish to skip the next chapter, the author of the Devil's Dictionary has some encouraging words:

"Abstainer—a weak person who yields to the temptation of denying himself a pleasure"
—Ambrose Bierce, 1911, American journalist

This contradicts the age-old truth as espoused in ancient Rome.

"Rule your mind, or it will rule you."
—Horace, Roman poet

CHAPTER SIX

DISCIPLINING THOUGHTS:
CONSEQUENCES OF ACTIONS

*"We all have our dreams. But in order to make dreams into reality,
it takes an awful lot of determination, dedication,
self-discipline and effort."*
—Jesse Owens, first black American Olympian, who shamed Hitler

Many religious leaders, after pondering the human condition, have gained insight into how our minds work. Practitioners of the arts of deep meditation in the Hindu and Buddhist traditions have added their own intuitions. Most start by recommending that you take a quiet moment to actually register what you are currently thinking about. This predated knowledge that thoughts were real things that could be recorded as actual electrical signals in your head.

Thinking about thinking, or becoming aware of one's thoughts, is important in realizing one's individuality. Cognition of our own participation and responsibility for events has helped mankind evolve over the past two thousand years. This helped bring about the understanding that the concept of "the Gods," or external forces, were responsible for every result in one's life was false. The monotheistic religions of the Middle East helped spur this trend in human thought by renouncing all other gods in favor of their chosen One. The modern idea and acceptance of individual responsibility for one's actions is thus relatively recent, coming late in the day after we began farming ten thousand years ago in the Tigris/Euphrates basin.

Yet even today, new linguistic research shows that some cultures retain the older legacy in their language in describing a misadventure. For example, an English newspaper might report "a man drove his car into a tree" with an understood substory that the man was to blame—drunk, going too fast for the bend, fighting with his wife in the car, on the cell phone, whatever. Or, conversely, the car manufacturer was at fault—bad brakes, faulty steering, malfunctioning gas pedal, or whatever the trial lawyers could dig up. Either way responsibility, and often attendant blame for not living up to that responsibility, would be assigned. In our world of torts there's money to be made from doing so, but it goes deeper than that.

A Japanese newspaper may report the very same misadventure as "the car hit the tree." Other languages and cultures likewise would omit reference to the man, and thus personal responsibility, from this accident. This is powerful stuff because it dissolves out of the description of the wreck any personal individual responsibility, avoiding it with the choice of words as their cultural norm.

So choice of words reflects on choice of thoughts, which recursively reflects on ways of thinking, and eventually, habits of acting. Punishment, a strong cultural enforcer, and definition of what constitutes a crime, thus derives differently depending on culturally different phrasing of events. Different cultures exist in part because they think differently than the way we think in our culture.

Buddhism advocates "gathering your stray thoughts." Jesuits, in their training, are asked to analyze each one of their thoughts during the preceding hour. Such mental discipline in these and other religions has helped lead to the conclusion that: "You are not responsible for the thoughts that enter your head, but you ARE responsible for the thoughts that you keep there."

Thus, self-discipline and awareness of your thoughts are a cornerstone in understanding how your self-help book works.

The ancient Chinese war strategist reflected on the potency of this awareness.

"Mastering others is strength, mastering yourself is power."
—Sun Tzu, *The Art of War*

The ancient Greeks got the message also:

"The first and best victory is to conquer self."
—Plato

This awareness of your thoughts gives you the luxury of replacing the dumb, stupid aberrant ones with the new goals and feelings that will help you triumph. In this, the self-help books are right, and worth their weight in gold for this advice. This permits the affirmations and visualizations described in later chapters to supplant your current disorganized mental chatter. To clean up the mess in your mental attic, your next self- discipline is as old as the bible and still valid today.

"And forgive us our trespasses,
as we forgive those who trespass against us"
—The Lord's Prayer, New Testament

Forgiveness is strongly advocated by all religions and most self-help books. This is because large amounts of conscious mental work—thinking—is just plain wasted or dissipated on negative emotions which form the laundry list of misery. We all get them so there's no shame in reiterating them: guilt, despair, loneliness, anger, lack, self-righteous indignation, justification, self-pity, limitation, revenge, desire for retribution, jealousy, envy, fear, resentment and frustration.

A glance at any daily newspaper or website readily shows the actions derived from the consequences of these thoughts, without the cleansing gift of forgiveness. If the list of negative emotions seems endless, it is because evolution has hard-wired them into our brains, reinforced by the prodding from the dark cellars of our limbic system in the lower recesses of our brains.

In past and present, the negative emotions and the actions they triggered served for societal coercion within the tribe or extended family. For those of you with families, this list may sound hauntingly familiar. From evolution's standpoint they conferred some survival value for the group, reducing dangerous behavioral transgressions within the group and solidifying the tribe against incursions from warring neighbors.

However, for the individual feeling them, obsessing over them, and pondering punitive actions, they become a severe constraint and drain on energies needed to focus on and take action to achieve personal goals. The darnedest thing is that they can be so satisfying and enjoyable! Commiserating friends with their concomitant attention over perceived wrongs constantly reinforce your accept-ance of negative feelings as normal, useful, natural, and indeed gratifying.

> *"Misery loves company."*
> —Old English proverb; says it all.

Forgiveness breaks the obsessive thought cycle. Letting go of past wrongs and perceived slights clears mental clouds for new thoughts. This is essential to permit space or neuronal function, for goal-oriented thoughts to flood the mind. This is what self-discipline is for. New thoughts and goals are the cardinal needs of self-help, inspiring hope instead of self-doubt and depression. Let me repeat that: awareness, cognizance or recognition of negative thoughts precedes forgiveness.

Training your mind to sound an alarm bell or hoist a red flag whenever negativity intrudes and takes over one's thinking is really tough at times. The negative thoughts often feel so right, the self-pity and wallowing in the past so socially expected and acceptable. Training over and over again to recognize these familiar feelings and flash on a new mental image can be learned. When practiced repeatedly until it becomes part of who you are, it can be joyously liberating.

This self-help discipline clears out the hot fires and ashes of vengeful thinking, with all that wasted drive and energy. It is necessary and essential if new thoughts of future achievements are to grow and take root in your mind. This can be undertaken in the steps your self-help books advocate. First: recognition that you are thinking negatively.

Second: replace it immediately with a positive image of desired results, as a conditioned response. Third: think through and feel forgiveness, both for yourself for past mistakes, and forgiving others that have "trespassed against you," to reinforce your new train of thought with your now-liberated mental muscle.

"We do not conquer the mountain, we conquer ourselves."
—Sir Edmund Hillary, first man to climb Mount Everest

Congratulations if you have already achieved this level of self-mastery and discipline over your thoughts. It will need to be revisited regularly. Thinking thus will become easier as you train or condition your mind to red-flag negative emotional clusters.

Dwelling on new desired results with bright mental images is very reinforcing, as it rewards you with the good feelings generated by a flood of neurochemicals surging through your brain's synapses.

"Little vicious minds abound with anger and revenge, and are incapable of feeling the pleasure of forgiving their enemies"
—Lord Chesterfield

What follows on from these exercises and successes is a renewed feeling of control, as your mind games begin to obtain you your desired personal improvement. Indeed, you do have more control. This sense of control is gratifying as you lick your thoughts into shape and watch and enjoy new results unfold from your actions. This, in turn, in a knock-on effect, enhances your self-esteem. You literally become and feel a better person.

"This self-help stuff really works," you say, as the feedback gives you the stamina and persistence to encourage you to stick with your program.

"If the brain sows not corn, it plants thistles."
—English proverb

With the removal of the crowding out of negative thoughts, your mind opens up for new visions and affirmations which we will explore later in this book. It may seem self-evidently obvious that without the active placement of *positive* thoughts in your mind— sowing corn—then thistles will grow in the empty wastelands, as the proverb above predicts. Actions springing from these thoughts are what you want to harvest to better your lot in life.

"As ye sow, so shall ye reap."
—Ephesians 6:5

Let us now examine, without too much psychological gobbledygook, the importance of your sense of self. Permit yourself to attend to the numerous facets of you, the personality of the "I" who looks back at you in the mirror each morning, and whom you create anew each waking minute.

"We all have a better guide inside ourselves, if we would attend to it, than any other person can be."
—Jane Austen

Your self-help book is there to encourage you—en-*courage*—or provide you with fresh courage, to change your sense of self and steer you toward a new triumphant you.

The tool they offer you is the words "I am...," adding whichever traits you aspire to.

This is an attempt to trigger alteration in your ego, that sense of self-identity to which you tightly cling and which you fervently believe is the "real" you. Although most self-help books preach humbleness as a means of quieting your ego, suppressing it with a mild self-effacing humility, you still need your ego to focus your sense of purpose. Your ego just has to be reprogrammed.

Much work has been done in this area, with the most infamous being the brainwashing of captured American soldiers by the Chinese during the Korean war and highlighted in the movie *The Manchurian Candidate.* Starting with small steps, the Chinese interlocutors got the American under indoctrination to agree to say "yes" to small things, such as "yes, the sun is shining outside today." Then they built on it with seemingly logical follow-ons until the man's entire belief system was transformed, turning him against his own country, which he was formerly willing to die for, and into a conforming communist supporter. This startlingly dramatic example of the plasticity of the sense of self-identity, with the acquirement of different mental faculties made necessary by the culture in which you survive, was foreseen and foretold over a century and a half ago by none other than Charles Darwin.

"In the distant future I see open fields for far more important researches. Psychology will be based on a new foundation, that of the necessary acquirement of each mental power and capacity by gradation."
—Charles Darwin, 1859, *The Origin of the Species*

The ability to let your old ego loosen its control over your daily life is necessary for you to impose your fresh new values. Relaxation of the old you permits you to forge a new ego and sense of enlarged possibilities with a different ego for yourself. The "I am" mantra of your self-help book is exquisitely powerful in this regard. Your ego is not immutable, and can be changed. The Pauline conversion of the cold and callous Saul on the road to Damascus into the generous and kind Saint Paul, evokes such an ego transformation as depicted in the Bible.

What's the problem, then? Why aren't we all transmutating ourselves into saints? Fear.

Fear of change. Our comfort zone starts acting up. Kicking and screaming like a child dragged away from his cake at a birthday party, your comfort zone yells out loud and clear: stop! Stop that right now! The butterflies in your tummy go haywire. You urgently need to find a toilet. Your self-help book spurs you on to become a different you, and your comfort zone lays it on thick: "Have you gone nuts trying to change? I'll show you who's in charge!" Guilt, unworthiness, self-doubt, recrimination, "I'm not good enough for that" feelings, anger, discouragement, and most of all fear hold us back.

Fear. The adrenaline pours into your bloodstream in that old familiar flight-or-fight response that necessarily kept your ancestors from becoming tiger food, and makes you feel so bloody awful!

Anything would feel better than the panic, the anxiety, the sheer misery eating away at your guts, and your mortifyingly atrocious self-talk and self-hate.

It's just too much to bear, and fifteen percent of us 300 million Americans gobble down anxiolytic benzodiazapines (Xanax, Valium, Ativan, etc.) each year to put a stop to the acting out of our comfort zones. Self-doubt is part of the human condition, holding us back from action.

"Our doubts are traitors, and make us lose the good
we oft might win by fearing to attempt."
—Shakespeare.

Whereas guilt can be finely honed by our culture

"Guilt—Jews are born with it, whilst Catholics have to learn it."
—Elaine Boozler, comedian

So how does your self-help book get you over this major hurdle? For if you are to change the results you want in your life, you have to work your way though it, and it can be so tough that some of us never make it, and live the rest of their lives lining the pockets of the benzodiazapines manufacturers. However, the comfort zone is never static; it grows and shrinks with new learning and fresh thoughts, or shrivels to a deathly embrace with slings and arrows of life's misfortunes. The alternative to challenging our comfort zone can be stifling as our poets warn us.

"He not busy being born is busy dying"
—Bob Dylan

Our psychologists admonish us to accept the pain and discomfort as a stark necessity for personal growth.

"There is no birth of consciousness without pain"
—Carl Jung

Easier said than done, Carl. Acceptance of the universal nature of this fear, unless you are a psychopath without care or conscience, helps ease the pain and helps us put a handle on it. It is, after all, energy, and adrenaline-fueled at that. We can use it, put it to good use. It is the very juice of life. The stage fright of the actor about to go on stage, or the rituals the surgeon uses to assuage his concealed excitement as he prepares to enter the operating room, reflects this energy surging through us.

Recognition of this need to change the self and alter the ego has not been missed by older cultures, as in the wise Indian admonition:

"If you want a place in the sun,
you must leave the shade of the family tree"
—Osage Indian proverb

Our more aggressive Navy SEAL training manual tells the troops to suck it up, and man up to the fears they must face every day in their world of dangerous action:

"Scared? You should be. But that's just your body's way of
saying it's alive. Now go to work."
Cannon & Cannon, SEAL Leadership Manual

This confrontation of one's own comfort zone and its zany fears is such a major hurdle that the self-help books keep trying to reassure us of its universality. Nevertheless, the brutal reality is that to achieve the new role model of the self you aspire to be and integrate it into your ego, you must remind yourself to take courage, believe you can, trust you can, and just do it.

"Life moves on, whether we act as cowards or heroes.
Life has no other discipline to impose, if we would but realize it,
than to accept life unquestioningly. Everything we shut our eyes to,
everything we run away from, everything we deny, denigrate or
despise, serves to defeat us in the end. What seems, nasty, painful,
evil, can become a source of beauty, joy and strength, if faced with
an open mind. Every moment is a golden one for him who has the
vision to recognize it as such."
—Henry Miller, Playwright

Creating this improved version of yourself relies on changing your thoughts, your beliefs about your capabilities, and ultimately all the new daily activities derived thereof.

" The ancestor of every thought is action."
—Emerson

Knowing which actions to take probably results more from your reprogrammed subconscious, or gut feeling, than your logical rational thoughts derived from your innate intelligence. Your self-help book helps you brainwash yourself with the mental tools and exercises laid out in these chapters. Consolidating new thoughts finally allows your subconscious to be consistent, and thus accept and pursue your newly chosen paths.

Although the self-help literature claims that thought alone can bring about your new reality, manifesting itself for you by focused intentions alone, the more pragmatic reader takes out the insurance of coupling it with new actions. These readers buy into the old folklore maxim: "If you keep on doin' what you've kept on doin', you goin' to keep on gettin' what you've been gettin'."

Or the lines of the ballad:

" Thinking and a-praying, wishing and a-hoping, planning and dreaming, won't get you into his heart."
—Burt Bacharach, sung by Dusty Springfield

Magic and miracles are the promise of some self-help texts. These help you manifest your heart's desires into consequences derived from new actions or opportunities. Ultimately, however, the endgame is for you to experience new and better feelings. The inexplicable cash windfall appearing suddenly in your life does what, exactly? Sure, you can eliminate those nagging debts, relieving feelings of guilt or fear of loss, and boost your self-esteem and pride. You can splurge on new possessions or a trip. However, most of the joy is in anticipation of buying, with the neurochemicals such as serotonin and dopamine that give you that shopping high dissipating from your brain synapses about one minute after your purchase. Though addictive, new shopping highs get harder and harder to achieve, and the thinking persons who pick up self-help tomes crave a more fulfilling life.

So how do we get motivated? What keeps us going? We are getting close to where the rubber hits the road with self-help, but it is here that evolutionary biology may for once hold us back. We all want the consequences, the results, of new habits that the new actions generate. But what's holding us back? Energy conservation is hard-wired into our biology by evolution. The couch-potato lifestyle always beckons. Its siren call to the weary is in continual conflict with the get-up-and-go needed to allow our humanity to blossom to its fullest potential. Your ability to overcome this yin/yang of alternating forces is where the self-help tools come in handy.

Belief, faith and trust must be instilled into the subconscious. This part of our mind must buy into your new self if it is to spur action persistently. Your job is to create a new mindset using the tools of faith and belief that are consistent with your existing neural pathways. The logical part of your mind craves consistency. The neural net algorithms being run in your brain may need it, not only to prevent dissonance, but also to actually function reliably. So how do you summon up belief? Logical thought helps, but it needs an emotional chaser. The biology of the brain needs limbic system input, some emotional feelings, to bolster belief. Faith is not a logical construct. Some turn to religion, finding the solemn belief of others imprinted in the written word is sufficient to fire up their juices, as in the classic:

> *"Ask and it will be given unto you; seek and ye shall find;*
> *knock and the door will be opened unto you."*
> —Matthew 7:7

Somehow this rendition in the old English words of the King James Bible resonate with some inner fire that punches up the written words with emotional impact. How this actually happens, is fertile ground for the neuroscientists seeking to unravel the biology that self-questioning triggers in your mind, because happen it does.

The tools of visualization and affirmation create new neural pathways impinging on your subconscious to create that feeling of certainty that embodies the sense of belief. Mentally rehearsed and repeated statements and mind movies bamboozle your brain into accepting your desired results as something real, tangible, possible, and even in your imagination as already in existence. Speaking out loud about your new paths is also advocated as a tool to consolidate your faith and belief in a changed reality. This mental training is what your self-help book is trying to teach you. New belief creates new habits of action as you strive toward your goals.

If your new way of thinking, your thoughts, are to have any real-life consequences, action is essential. The words of one guru of the self-help tribe could not be more explicit:

> *"Often the difference between a successful man and a failure is not one's better abilities or ideas, but the courage on has to bet on his ideas, to take a calculated risk—and to act."*
> —Maxwell Maltz, plastic surgeon, author of *Psychocybernetics*

Betting on ideas first presupposes clear-cut, well-defined goals. Asking yourself what it is you really, really want out of life is often the first step away from muddled thinking, on a journey to self-fulfillment. Goals also set belief more firmly in your subconscious, as logical action steps spring from explicit goals, and your subconscious recognizes action as something real and true. Goals help you turn the invisible into the visible, manifesting your desires.

Gratitude, and feeling good and happy, is suggested by the self-helps as shortcuts to the mental hygiene necessary to incorporate faith and belief into your mind. Humor and laughter are constant companions on life's path in cleansing the negativity which precludes new thought and action. This advice is not restricted to the self-helps, but found in religious texts and the musing of politicians.

> *"He deserves paradise who makes his companion laugh."*
> —The Koran

> *"Life is short. Live it up."*
> —Nikita Khrushchev

Laughter and the act of gratitude, saying thank you for all the many blessings in life which you already enjoy, cannot co-exist with the negative rantings of an upset comfort zone. Your old yin/yang tension exists, and only one group of emotions can win. When your self-help book exhorts you to bring feelings into the equation of your self re-programming, it is the positive ones you need, not the negativity. On a simple practical level, a smiling happy face attracts more cooperation from others than a scowl. The social lubricant of saying "thank you" provides for more gracious human interaction and, perhaps cynically, yet even more cooperation that can be used to go for the gold.

Still and yet, the old energy-preserving evolutionary biology pops up and upsets the apple cart by demanding, why bother? Why subject yourself to the burdensome tasks of awareness, thought changing, deleting negativity, forgiveness, ego modification, expressing gratitude, affirming, visualizing, evincing joy, goal-setting and all the rest?

You could just go down to the pub and sup a pint. The non-achievers will just try and drag you down anyway, as you are starting to show them up as slackers. Apart from self-respect, there is that nagging little feeling like a stone in your shoe, that perhaps, just perhaps mind you, let's not get carried away, maybe there is something more, a better life awaiting jut around the corner. As we only get one chance, one go around in this life, what a devastating loss to miss it. As one surgeon puts it perhaps a bit grimly:

"The reason you strive in life to learn, change, grow and improve yourself daily is because the alternative is so bleak: a closed mind with unchanging ignorance condemning you to a stale rut, ending your days as a relic of bygone times, a has-been with your potential extinguished, awaiting your grave."
—Christopher Lyon, oculofacial surgeon, 2001

CHAPTER SEVEN

CHOICE

"Choices are the hinges of destiny."
—Pythagoras

Choice, the act of choosing one's thoughts and making a decision, is paramount in all your self-help manuals. Even the act of not choosing, indecision, is a choice. There is nothing you have to do; everything is a choice, beautifully put in the old Spanish saying:

"Choose what you want, said God: then pay the price."
—Spanish proverb

You can have anything you want, but you can't have everything you want because you only have so much time. You have to choose. So perhaps Mick Jagger was closer to the mark in his song:

"You can't always get what you want."
—The Rolling Stones

In contradistinction to the mundane practicalities of the previous chapter on thought discipline and beginning actions, choice may reflect a quantum mechanical brain event, described by physicists as "collapse of the wave function potential." This esoteric concept is based on the notion that our universe has a multitude of potential possibilities that, in some models, all exist at the same time. In a seemingly magical fashion, the act of human choice, observation or thought forces our brain to select one of these possibilities, and the rest disappear.

Amazingly, by extension of this theory, enslaved by the inexorable logic of their mathematical equations, some scientists argue that human choices expressed in thought have actually shaped and determined the universe we live in. Each act of observation in their theory collapses entire ranges of possibilities and selects just one, with each step leading ultimately to the universe we now live in. Our world, in our universe, results from our thoughts that have become manifest in reality. The astonishing implications of these theories caused the gentle Einstein to complain that "God did not play dice with the universe."

Even more astounding to the lay mind is the proposition that the mathematics of quantum theory permit these effects to run forward in time. The physicists have a weasel escape clause when it comes to time. It is not the time that you and I enjoy, with birth and death and some down time at the beach in the middle. Oh no, either time does not exist in their calculus, or it all exists at once and we perceive changes as an illusion. Moreover, in their figurings, time can run forward and backward. So, because they are smarter than the rest of us, we may just have to accept their non-human precepts, which do not fit in to our day-to-day experiences of morning, noon and night, and if we are lucky, a paycheck at the end of the week.

Let us explore another aspect of this conjecture that ultimately reflects your human choice. An additional esoteric effect is at play in creating our universe the way we like it, so to speak. Events occur in steps. Each step either forward or backward in time embraces a gazillion possibilities. These possibilities can be impacted by human thought, with choices made on what to focus on being under human control.

Thought, being a real electromagnetic event in the universe, impacts the cloud of possibilities that engulf each step, going either forward or backward in time. This thought acts as an observation, a physical engagement, with the multitude of possibilities which favors that possibility being focused on.

This adds new relish to the old saying "be careful what you wish for, you might get it." The other possibilities lose whatever energy they possessed, and all shrivel away like the Wicked Witch of the West in the *Wizard of Oz*, leaving behind the one event envisioned and encapsulated in our thoughts. Well, if that's not scary, what is?

The esoteric effect is embodied in a concept gloriously termed "the inverse Zeno phenomenon" that can be best understood as follows. If a possibility even exists, no matter by how many steps removed in the future, inverse Zeno allows that if this future possibility becomes acknowledged as a thought, which we now know is a real electromagnetic entity, then it can become manifest in reality. What's more, it is favored when stacked against all other entities because of the energy and information contained within the thought. Even more incredible, the inverse Zeno can draw or propel events in a series of steps, even when the thought is *many steps ahead* of the current starting point.

Formulae are the death knell for any author's hopes of book sales, but this point is so important to our understanding of how choice impacts our universe, that I beg you to bear with me.

In the inverse Zeno dynamic, events enfold in a series of steps, labeled A, B, C, D, etc. As in A > B >C > D >E, then if human thought imagines or conjures up the thought that 'E' could exist, or would be desirable, then the other events or properties A, B, C, D, which may also *not* exist at present, could be retroactively brought into being!

The very thought of E being real feeds back the possibility of D being real, and more probable to be selected out of the cloud of possibilities. Now the retroactive chain reaction of possibilities appears to flow backwards in time, with D's existence now stimulating, promoting and inducing the existence of C and all the others likewise.

Thus, A<B<C<D <<< E*—thought *.

This induction by inverse Zeno permits the concrete real event to unfold and happen in the normal sequence we expect to see in our common sense, non-magical world experience.

Does thinking really make it so? Well, this presupposes one elegant, beautiful thought sitting there all alone like a fairy-tale princess in all her glory, in total isolation from the roar of the freeway traffic blasting past her castle window. Noise exists, get over it, Princess! Nevertheless, this mechanism is thought by many physicists to be a real possibility consistent with the quantum theory, regardless of the noise of the constant buzz of energies that drench our minds and flood our planet.

Thoughts can become manifest in reality, just as our self-help book maintains, and now there is even a plausible mechanism to account for it. If we can conceive it, pathways, steps or channels open up in a retrograde (to our human mind's perception of time) fashion to manifest it preferentially into being. Hard for our caveman brains to grasp, I agree, but there is more than one physicist who claims this to be true.

As difficult as this may be to follow, it's the foundation and essence of positive thinking, affirmation and visualizations so frequently taught in the self-help books. Let us try and comprehend this incredible story from physics. A thought—your thought—is a real electromagnetic event in your head that can be detected with appropriate detectors above your scalp. Our universe is abuzz with myriads of potential possibilities, and some claim myriad *universes*, with zillions of pathways leading to these possible events or properties. A choice, the thought you decide to retain in your mind and focus on, a persistent thought, better still one larded up with your strongest heartfelt emotions, fixes one outcome out of a multitude of future possibilities.

The bizarre concept that the universe was created for our benefit, as the conditions are just perfect for the emergence of man and thought, is no longer a religious tenet as espoused in the Bible. Scientists are aware that if any of a number of the universe's conditions and physical constants were just a shade off, our existence would not have been possible. Our biology would never have been created, and because of this our human friendly universe has been christened "anthropomorphic," or designed for human life.

The anthropomorphic universe model in some of its iterations has been explained by the very same inverse Zeno effects that have been used to explain manifestation of thoughts. Simply put, because we are here our very existence precludes all other possibilities, and as such exerts a retrograde influence on the probabilities of all the necessary steps and conditions in the universe that would prevent our existence, and establishes the prerequisites to ensure that we did evolve.

This sounded like circular reasoning the first time I read it, too. I got hung up on my biological background, arguing that the universe is fifteen *billion* years old, yet humanoid-type critters have only been around since the Ardi-Lucy eon of four to seven *million* years ago, so how could thought induce anything older, prior to the organisms that evolved to possess thought itself?

It's the age/time thing again. I was thinking like a normal time-enmeshed human being, instead of the liberated physicist for whom time is just another function in his equations. Beyond all common reason and sense, the equations of those who posit the anthropomorphic model universe being drawn into being by inverse Zeno steps by our emphatically human presence allow the Zeno phenomenon to extend all the way back to the Big Bang, and perhaps even beyond. Of course, this is altogether staggeringly mind-blowing to us mere mortals. But it is included here in this book, exploring self-help mechanisms of thought projection and involvement in creating aspects of our universe and lives, to permit your mind to expand to some of the far-out (pun intended) scientific theories out there.

Fixing the outcome of random possibilities by choice of thought and observation is a classic experiment in quantum physics that has been repeated in many labs throughout the world. It is an accepted fact. Your thought does this by its very existence; its chosen retention by you from all your other mental clutter emanates a powerful focus. Because your thought now exists, its resonance can exert retrograde influence, enhancing pathways back to your present condition. This makes it more likely to happen, its statistical odds improved over other possibilities. Your thought is inducing itself into real expressed existence. It manifests itself. You have moved from the relatively intangible, unseeable thought to a concretely expressed event. Your self-help book has encouraged, cajoled and enabled you along this path.

Thoughts do not occur in isolation from other activities. Most importantly, from a statistical perspective, the first *action* towards a goal dramatically increases the odds of movement towards a new goal. This seems like common sense, but a deeper underlying reality in following Zeno's steps is also at play, whether we realize it or not. Perhaps Dr. King had some inkling of this dual quality of the practical, coupled with an act of will recruiting the powers of the mind's thought when he made his astute observation:

"Take the first step in faith; you don't have to see the whole staircase."
—Martin Luther King Jr.

Choice at the practical, functioning, prosaic level is well put by the famous athlete:

"There aren't many clearly marked signpost moments in your life,
but occasionally they do come along, and you have a choice.
You can either do something the same old way, or you can make
a better decision. You have to be able to recognize the moment,

and to act on it, at the risk of saying later 'That's when it all could have been different'."
—Lance Armstrong, cyclist

Choice, what we select to think about, is clearly linked to goals. It is human nature to strive for such.

"Man is a goal seeker."
—Aristotle

Should the quantum physicists and neuroscientists get together on the same page and confirm this remarkable feat of human will, creating a universe no less if you buy into their arguments, the results and conclusions will be monumental in scope. New Agers may believe this already without the arduous research demanded by serious science, but the bulk of the population needs hard factual evidence, and rightly so, before it concedes this to be true.

Acceptance by the general population will mean that mental hygiene will be taught in school. Recognition and discarding of negative thoughts, although of some survival value to the tribe for group cohesion, will find its place in the syllabus, under the protests of both the civil libertarians and conservative free-thinkers. Replacing negative thoughts with positive ones that unlock our human potential will be the order of the day.

Accolades already are assigned to visionaries like the crusty old Yorkshireman, Arthur C. Clarke, who put forth the concept of earth-circling satellites and taught us that:

"Any sufficiently advanced technology is indistinguishable from magic"
—Arthur C. Clarke, sci-fi writer

Whereas we shudder at how human minds could conceive the ovens at Dachau.

What are the consequences for the human race, rejoicing at the lunar landings and all that huge milestone entails, versus dwelling on such horrors as the Khmer Rouge's Tuol Sleng prison? The left-wing mind bending in the salons at the Sorbonne in Paris filled the minds of the Khmer Rouge's leaders, leading step by inexorable step to the emptying of the capital city's Phnom Penh population into the meat grinder of the Cambodian killing fields. Thoughts have consequences. From moon to stinking rice paddy, regardless of the actual mechanism, both these opposite poles of human activity first began in the minds of men, as thoughts. Then they happened.

> *"We are what we think. All that we are arises with our thoughts.*
> *With our thoughts we make the world."*
> *"What we think, we become."*
> —Buddha

CHAPTER EIGHT

AFFIRMATIONS

"I think, therefore I am."
—Descartes

Your self-help book would rephrase this, still maintaining the cardinal three P's of Present tense, Positive tone and Personal statement, as: "I am, therefore I think."

The concept behind how this tool works for you is to establish your focus on the positive, supplanting whatever negative thoughts are running untrammeled through your mind. Repetition through verbalization uses your conscious mind. It accepts it as true and real when the personal pronoun "I" is used in the present tense, becoming integrated into your ego or sense of self.

This is accomplished by its acceptance into your subconscious, where it integrates into your belief system as a deep conviction. Once installed in your subconscious as a conviction, your mind goes on to automatic and begins to express your conviction in your daily actions, and move you towards your desired goals.

An example would be a recovering convalescent healing from a painful ankle injury repeating to himself, "I am getting fitter and fitter each and every day. I'm getting fitter and fitter in each and every way."

Note that this complies with the requirements of personal, present tense and positive outlook. When coupled with self-imagery of the man with his ankle fully restored, functional and healed, it conforms to Leonardo da Vinci's advice of asking questions as to your desired result, then working backwards in the steps needed to attain it.

This is all sound, prosaic, self-evident, practical advice, but it is amazing how few of us are taught to use it, and must first encounter it in our self-help book, rather than in our school education. Having covered the basics, which require none of the esoteric physics encountered in the last chapter, let us examine other ways in which self-help books assist you in achieving your heart's desires.

We all bring mental baggage into adulthood, and your self-help books work by pointing the way to overcome our fears and self-doubts. No one, no matter how successful, vain, arrogant, or self-confident, gets through his week without a whisper from his mental nagging apparatus (and we are not talking about the wife), even if it's just a question of, "How can I can I become even better at what I'm doing?"

This anxiety, heebie-jeebies or fear springs from the older parts of our brain dealing with emotions, the limbic system, near the base of our skull. The old cliché that we are now here and alive because of fear remains true. Fear of that rustling in the bushes warned our cavemen ancestors so they did not end up as tiger food. It still keeps us from stepping into the road in front of a truck (even scientists who declare we have no free will, that our lives are all pre-ordained), and reminds us to lock our doors at night.

It hones our survival skills, with fears from our ancestral memories of poisonous creatures like spiders and snakes, even though most of them are more afraid of you than you are of them. Logic and intelligence alone could not confer this survival protection.

Like it or not, we are stuck with the yin/yang of emotion versus reason. Intellect and passion, constantly vacillating and regrouping, is what makes us human. Elections are often won more based on emotional feelings for a candidate or his opponent, than the cold, calculating clear-headedness of the early morn, when our minds are refreshed with neurotransmitters, recharged from a good night's sleep.

So thoughts of worthlessness, guilt, self-pity, anger, revenge, retribution, resentment, fear, justification, jealousy and all the rest will continue to well up in us and swirl through our thoughts for as long as the human race shall be. Getting all these toys back in the box under the bed before Mother storms in is your job, as your self-help book unfailingly advises.

Nowhere is this constant interplay between opposite poles of human behavior better displayed than the hormone oxytocin, which is secreted by the pituitary-hypothalamus part of the brain, and the heart and other blood vessels in the body. Oxytocin has a Jekyll and Hyde effect on the body. It normally is associated with "good" effects such as uterine contractions during labor and milk let-down in the nursing mother. In the latter, oxytocin release during nursing creates a pleasant dreamy state that is thought to encourage bonding with the infant and reward the brain for the activity of breast feeding.

Interestingly, oxytocin, also known as the trust hormone, helps boost social skills in autistic adults, overcoming their in built reticent shyness. This bonding effect is seen in many mammals, resulting from oxytocin release that creates a warm afterglow for lovers after love-making. It earned the nickname the "cuddle hormone." However, the soap operas and trashy romance novels bear stark testimony to the capricious uncertainty of the reliability of oxytocin's cuddle effect following human intercourse. This inconstancy in infallibly inducing bonding reflects differences between the sexes, diminishment with age, genetic differences and the tug of all the other daily events that enswirl us.

But there is more to this story, more fodder for the purple prose sheets and soap operas. Oxytocin has a dark side. In addition to the feel-good cuddle effects that stimulate pair bonding, evolution has used oxytocin as a tool to cement the bond even further, with the very negative emotions of jealousy, resentment, rage and envy. The movie *Fatal Attraction* could well be the very best showpiece of this dark side of oxytocin's reach into the human psyche.

The movie's main female character (with apologies to the ladies, it often seems to affect them more than men as they release higher quantities of oxytocin than the male, but male stalkers and jealous rage show that men are not immune) pursues her chosen mate with a clingy, needy vigor that reflects precious little love, and an overwhelming boiling rage of envy, anger and jealous resentment.

Oxytocin, love it and hate it. Happy couples get lucky if they can enjoy oxytocin's cuddle effects without the downside of *Fatal Attraction's* brutal venom. Careers in marriage counseling are built on managing this yin/ yang in human affairs.

Of course, the Bard noted this with his uncanny perception of human nature, centuries ago in jolly old England.

> *"Hell hath no fury like a woman scorned."*
> —Shakespeare

Affirmations help supplant negative feelings with more useful thoughts on a more automatic basis than the chores of casting about for awareness of negative thinking, red-flagging the troublemaker, and popping a happy image into the toaster. Repetition, and some self-help books push for one thousand verbalizations an hour, helps your affirmation burrow down deep into your subconscious. With training and practice, affirmations compel themselves to be expressed in actions, as we identify ourselves with the new traits.

This degree of persistence may overwhelm your brain, and may in fact be unnecessary. Changes in the brain's short-term memory clearinghouse, the hippocampus, have been observed with just four repetitions per hour. After processing, memory is thought to be shunted to the long-term memory stores in the lower brain temporal lobes for a more permanent home entwined in the neuronal DNA. Naps, as reviewed elsewhere, help this shunting process, so that affirmations repeated before sleep may stand a better chance of "taking" than affirmations made during the maelstrom of your day's activities. However, do not let this discourage you if you suffer from a swamp of negativity. Then, by all means, if a positive affirmation breaks the stranglehold of miserable thoughts, use it as often as need be.

"If you want a quality, act as if you already had it.
Try the 'as if' technique."
—William James, psychologist

Fresh action, derived from our affirmations, with a willingness, even compulsion, to be consistent in who we feel ourselves to be, is what brings about the changes our self-help book promises. The self-discipline imposed by replacing our brooding pet peeves with an often contrary self-affirmation gives birth to our underused abilities. In and of itself, this self-discipline is salutatory in establishing better habits and work ethics that increase our productivity. Synergism is found in the associated increase in self-esteem that is a corollary of these efforts.

"Trust yourself. Create the kind of self that you will be happy to live
with all your life. Make the most of yourself by fanning the tiny,
inner sparks of possibility into flames of achievement."
—Golda Meir

Affirmations do require constant repetition, because the coherent quantum states of your goal thoughts rapidly dissipate into decoherence as the overwhelming mass of other mental activities and neurochemical events concurrently happening in your brain as you live your life quickly dwarf the puny signal of your will or goal thought.

The cardinal affirmation is the present tense "I AM…" This personal ideal is picked up by the subconscious ego or self-identity. If repeated with enough frequency and emotional intensity, strengthened by a fervid belief in its truth—the "act as if" of William James—then over time it will be incorporated into you, your newly adopted you, your shiny new self.

Your ego strives for logical consistency. Once your affirmation, such as "I am a non-smoker with clean, healthy, athletic lungs," finally becomes incorporated into your subconsciously held belief in who you are, your actions *must* reflect these new innate concepts. Deeds, such as lighting up a cigarette, now will lie outside the realm of your newly affirmed self, and it will feel uncomfortable or even impossible for you to enact, as if you had undergone self-hypnosis, which in a way you have. You will have now completed your transformation. This is how your self-help book works.

Notwithstanding the potency of repeated affirmations, they lack the beefed up power of questions. Questions that you persistently ask yourself, change your mental concentration. Questions bring focus, alter your thoughts and thus change your behavior in more powerful steps than affirmations alone. New thoughts are grabbed with emotional hooks put out by your limbic system. These thoughts now linked with emotion, spur action that gets you different results.

Your self-help books strongly admonish you not to ask the multiverse *how* you can achieve your goals, but rather to just trust, intend, expect and anticipate with faith, which may well indeed work. Regardless of the fact that this tactic may achieve results, asking *yourself* questions will always reliably refocus your thoughts triggering acts that bring you closer to your goals.

"If you haven't got anything nice to say about anybody,
come sit next to me."
—Alice Roosevelt Longworth

Humans gossip. Although Biblical injunction against giving false witness is embedded in its commandments for social order and peace, most folks recognize that gossip oils the gears of social intercourse. We are all familiar with the re-hashing over and over of some social slight to any willing listener. Balzac, a prolific French writer of the early 1800s, was also a keen detective of human nature who observed:

"When it comes to minor affairs of life,
one has to go into a great deal of detail."
—Balzac

Male chauvinism does not preclude the reality that the female is more loquacious than the male, with a quicker tongue and more to say than the hapless male, who struggles to arrange his linear thinking, edit responses for tact, eliminate *faux pas* and invariably ponderously thinks up his retort five minutes after the conversation has ended!

Perhaps that is why so many authors are male, as writing gives them time to put their thoughts in order, presenting them on paper in a fashion they could never achieve in a timely manner in a give-and-take with the female. Of course, male lawyers, comedians and politicians, which some would say unkindly are all the same, make their very livings by overcoming this male handicap.

So, if we can accept that the female has honed gossip to an art form, perhaps we can tease out more readily its social functions from their exemplary display and learn how this may redound to the art of self-help. The obvious roles of female gossip are embodied in the performance of the five "E"s: Explore, Enhance, Enable, Exhort and finally Enforce social mores, as seen from the female's evolutionary perspective. Nibbling away like acid at someone else's self-esteem, prestige and hence privilege serves the function of demoting the aberrant rival female, thus elevating the relative position of the gossiping female within her social group. What's a girl to lose? And it's good juicy fun into the bargain!

Another common thread is present in gossip that reflects on one's sense of self-worth and its power, utilized to good effect in the affirmation technology of your self-help book. The intense reflective sifting and parsing of every tiny morsel, to mine and leach out the very last drop of meaning from an encounter and its conversation, entrances the gossipers, seeming endlessly. Why is this so?

What other purpose is served by searchingly rooting out every last detail, as Balzac would have it, into "the minor details of life?" This is where both male and female converge. There is a strongly felt need for justification, for validation that one was "right" in the encounter under discussion. The need for human reassurance from your listener that you did and said the correct things reflects the deeply felt disturbance that the encounter provoked in your comfort zone.

One's sense of self, or ego, was under attack, and this challenge to who we believe ourselves to be cannot go unanswered. Hence the dredging up again and again of every irritating and aggravating facet until our bruised ego is calmed, pacified and settled, like a colicky baby that demands soothing attention.

Your self-help books direct the construction of one's ego or sense of self with affirmations, tapping in to this incredible power and enormous need for vindication, justification and validation. The repetitive affirmative act of proclaiming to yourself over and over "I AM a healthy non-smoker (or whatever qualities you desire to possess)" in the present tense, seeks to engage and integrate your desired quality into that part of your mind that constitutes your ego. Once locked in there, with newly constructed neural pathways in your brain, it becomes your new comfort zone. You have expanded it. You will feel an irresistible compunction, an obligatory compulsion to express and demonstrate this new quality whenever the need arises in your new life.

Assisting you in maintaining internal consistency, you now have the support of a newly subconsciously accepted personality trait that you have conned yourself into believing with your affirmations. You no longer have to struggle and strive to showcase your new habit, as it automatically has become part of you, exuding itself under compulsion whenever life's challenges present, indicating that it really is now a component of your current self-identity.

"The thing always happens that you really believe in: and the belief in a thing makes it happen."
—Frank Lloyd Wright

So, affirmations made passionately with intense emotion and belief, repeatedly, do work. They change who you were into who you want to be. Your doubts may be assuaged as your self-help books are right; they have latched onto an underlying truth and cannot be dismissed as bogus charlatanry, insofar as affirmations produce results.

The raw recruit who at first may not perceive himself as a warrior, after the repeated indoctrination, education and training of boot camp, reinforced by wearing his uniform, particularly back into his former home environment, and shooting his gun with his comrades in arms, begins to identify and express himself as a soldier. With this intense immersion, the new soldier may never consciously recognize his own affirmations. In casual conversations with former friends and family his uniform will speak volumes, but when asked he will respond "I am a soldier." The conversion is complete.

And so it is with you, when you embark alone on your journey of self-improvement. Some of the affirmations you may use as a tool may be so self-evidently obvious, such as "I am a tech student," that they will be uttered without stress or strain, requiring little if any emotional intensity. Major transformative goals may likewise be achieved as your follow the normal progression through college to graduation and job, with cursory attention to the affirmations of who you are becoming. It is the challenges of life, the forks in the road, the rainy days, that will require the power of your amped-up affirmations to resolve.

Focus is honed by affirmations. They generate and promote curious questions centered on results. Dwelling on results replaces brooding over pet peeves as your conscious brain responds to the newly inculcated affirmations and sense of self. Repeated focus on new and fresh results energizes and enables new habits to develop and emerge, often rapidly, amazing both yourself and your friends. Novel deeds begin.

"The journey of ten thousand miles begins with a single phone call."
—Confucius Bell

Your newly affirmed self can assert itself with a seemingly effortless, miraculous and robust vigor. Yes, affirmations can, and do, work well.

CHAPTER NINE

VISUALIZATION

"The eye and the brain are not like a fax machine,
nor are there little people looking at the images coming in."
—Thorsten Wiesel, Nobel laureate and vision neurophysiologist

The Marine who practices disassembly and reassembly of his rifle inside a cloth bag has certainly trained himself in this battlefield survival skill by his use of touch and feel. However, he cannot see inside the darkened bag. This soldier must *visualize* his gun's parts, where they slide apart and where they click together. He forms an image of the assembled gun in his mind's eye to guide him through the necessary steps. Bullets go in one end, the barrel at the other. In the pitch darkness of a night raid, if his rifle falls in the mud he can clean it and make it serviceable again. It can make the difference for him of returning home a victorious hero, or in a body bag.

Our brain's ability to form images is one of life's glorious miracles. Self-help books draw heavily on this biological wonder to reprogram, or in most instances to *initiate* a program, that will move you towards the goals and results you seek. Even the most mundane day to day vision is a triumph and marvel of evolution.

We awaken. We open our sleepy eyes. Those of us lucky enough to enjoy pleasant dreams with vistas of sunny tropical isles find these dream images immediately replaced by the familiar "real" features of our bedroom. The alarm clock, the sunlight peeping through the geometrical regularity of our window shutters, the end of our bed covers, all flood instantaneously into our sensorium, swamping and obliterating our dream visions.

But in a sense, our waking "real" vision is also a dream. It is created not from grains of silver salts like photographic film, or electronic pixels of your phone's digital camera, that all fuse to create a picture with the illusion of reality like an impressionist painting, but from a mundane collection of about six different elements that reside in the retinas at the back of our eyeballs.

Our vision is created from such mundane sensors or detectors as edges, movement, different light wavelengths that we perceive as colors, contrast differences, and vertical, horizontal or oblique orientations. Visible light makes up about one-billionth of the electromagnetic spectrum, yet we have evolved to let it account for, and be, our whole visual world.

This mish-mash of different electromagnetic signals detected by specialized retinal cells is partially ordered and catalogued in our retinas before being shunted as electrical nerve impulse signals into our optic nerves, both of which penetrate our skulls behind our eyeballs, cross over and spread out in a highly organized fashion along the side of our brains, ending up near the back of our skulls in a region termed the occipital cortex.

About one-third of our brain is given over to processing our vision, so evolution values it highly, as our brains consume about twenty percent of the energy from our food intake.

Guess what? There is no IMAX screen back there. There is no movie projector, no TV screen, no little man watching all that's going on out there in the real world. So what's really going on, and how does it impact the visualization rituals so heavily promulgated by our self-help books?

We imagine it. Everything. The beautiful colors, the dreamy swooping curves of your new car, the aesthetic masterpiece of the male form of David by Michelangelo, Google images of earth, spacemen kicking up dust on the moon, the arresting curves and declivities of the nubile female nude, and the sheer artistry of the simplest flower, all are constructs of our imagination.

Our pictorial image construction is an illusion made up from the firing of nerve impulses along axons, with the release of neurotransmitters at synapses in our brain that create hovering and penetrating wave forms which we interpret as the magic of vision. Sight, as perceived, defies explanation with our limited vocabulary.

Although we are hamstrung in our ability to fully understand and explain the pictures our brains generate, we can, and certainly do, use them. Conjuring up images in our imagination (which is mostly visual, as one would expect from this word's root: "to form images") enables our childhood brains to grow and mature.

Forward planning, whether a shopping expedition, military planning or a Martian landing, all benefit from visualization. Surgeons, athletes and actors all review pictures in their heads to practice their moves beforehand. It is second nature to us all and part of what makes us human, as we can share words in conversation that bring up similar images in our mind's eyes, that enable, enrich, facilitate and generate interest in any discussion or dialogue.

> *"When I'm ready to take a photograph I quite obviously*
> *see in my mind's eye something that is not literally there...*
> *I'm interested in something which is built up from within,*
> *rather than just extracted from without."*
> —Ansel Adams, photographer

The term "mind's eye" was invented by the visionary Shakespeare, who added hundreds of new words to the English language, and in our context, intriguingly used it to describe a ghost in Hamlet. Our mental images are indeed ephemeral and ghost-like, but serve us well nevertheless when we develop a new skill such as a golf swing, or a mental map of highways to arrive at your favorite shopping mall (although the latter visualization is sadly and rapidly becoming an obsolescent skill, with the advent of GPS map screens in our cars).

Your self-help book advocates and teaches you to optimize this visualization skill, applying it to achieving your desired goals. Most of us do it already on a regular basis.

> *"A couple of times a day I sit quietly and visualize my body*
> *fighting the AIDS virus. It's the same as me sitting and seeing*
> *myself hit the perfect serve. I did that often as an athlete."*
> —Arthur Ashe, tennis player

So you have grasped the basic technique of visualization and some of the underlying science. You understand that repeatedly imagining yourself in the illusory cinema of your mind, actively and vividly achieving some set goal, increases the recruitment of nerve pathways and synapses, developing new, stronger neural pathways to reinforce your subconscious mindset. Your goals can be outrageous, but now your visualizations have given you a new confidence to persist. As Churchill saw it:

> *"The most absurd aspirations have sometimes led*
> *to extraordinary success."*
> —Winston Churchill

The ice skater's triple jump, or the racetrack driver's slide through the curves, are all rehearsed over and over in mental pictures until they become as natural as tying your shoe laces or brushing your teeth. Your mental pictures become indistinguishable from reality.

Well, practice makes perfect, you protest, what's so special about visualization? Pilots use flight simulators to simulate engine flameout at 36,000 feet. Young surgeons practice their skills on cadavers, embedding the three-dimensional anatomy in their memories, so that when the knife is put to warm, bleeding, living flesh, they can make their cuts unerringly. Yet this is not visualization, although it is obviously involved, as the other senses of touch and feel of their instruments, and response to their actions, provides instantaneous tactile feedback for their training and incorporation into their memory banks.

But is that all there is to it, you may ask? Is it all just a head game, as a prelude to rolling up your sleeves and getting down to work? Is it just a mild confidence booster that provides you with the juice to persist through obstacles and frustration? This prosaic and mundane worldview appears to be shared by some of the world's success stories, as in the remarks of the comic actor Jim Carrey:

"I would visualize things coming to me. It would just make me feel better. Visualization works if you work hard. That's the thing. You just can't visualize and go eat a sandwich."
—Jim Carrey

You may have noted that, contrary to your self-help book's admonition to feel good whilst visualizing, Jim states clearly that he did it to *make* him feel better. However, you now know that visualization is an exquisitely powerful and useful tool that taps into your brain's inherent imaging system, using the very same pathways that you use in everyday vision. Your sight depends on your imagination to create an illusion, and you use the very same imagination to conjure up your visualization images, so that your brain cannot distinguish between what is real or illusory, and it is always an illusion anyway.

Your self-help book is rightly proud of including visualization in its program as it serves to push aside energy wasting negative thoughts and emotions, enforcing focus on desired goals, and representing one of the most astounding examples of mental self-discipline. Of all the tools, it comes closest to creating belief. Confidence springs from belief. When your belief becomes enacted into factual reality that you can see, touch, feel and experience the results thereof, you have entered into the realm of and transited to faith. Tangible results reward and reinforce faith. A feedback cycle of trust in yourself has been born, and the spillover to your self-esteem energizes you to tackle bigger and better projects, speeding up your movement towards accomplishing your desires. Religions have preached belief, trust, hope and faith for generations. Now you have the tools to individually achieve them. You have power.

> *"Hope springs eternal in the human breast."*
> —Alexander Pope

The tantalizing carrot of mysticism is held forth by many self-help books when it comes to visualization, hinting, or boldly proclaiming that you can stage-manage your own future using this technique. The suggestion being that your brain is interacting with the universe with its mental images of the future to help manifest it into reality above and beyond the humdrum practice of your imagination.

If this is so, it would invoke the inverse Zeno effect explained elsewhere in this book. Should this be indeed in operation, a mental image backed with a fierce emotional punch would project a lot more information out there into the universe than the single thought discussed previously. By the image's very existence it would collapse other possible future images, thus actively selecting your desired goal from all others, and set in train the enhanced probability of the sequence of steps necessary for its enactment in a retrograde fashion. It might be expected to be a more powerful inducer than a single thought, by virtue of all its additional information, making your self-help's visualization one of its most powerful devices in its toolbox.

CHAPTER TEN

TIME, GENTLEMEN PLEASE

Our caveman ancestors knew about electromagnetic radiation. They experienced the warmth that could peel their skins from that fireball of continuous nuclear explosions in the heavens, our sun. Light shone in the morning and went away at night. Sound waves were important for finding food and avoiding danger, when alert to a snake's hiss or predator's roar.

The rhythmic slap of waves on a shoreline meant food in the form of shellfish and cockles and mussels alive, alive oh. Our migrations out of Africa followed the coastlines of Arabia fed by fish caught from the waves of the littoral zone. The populating of the Americas over thirteen thousand years ago traced from the Bering land bridge down the shores of the Pacific coast, evidenced by prehistoric shellfish middens on the Channel Islands off Santa Barbara.

Sound and infrared waves pleasantly intermingled as our caveman sheltered in his cave, enjoying his scavenged meat, or occasional fellow human, roasting on the flames of his fire. Whilst snugly ensconced he listened to the sounds of the sighing wind soughing at his cave mouth, or the sounds of winter gales rattling the last leaves off the trees.

Gravity too was understood by our caveman. Gravity ensured that something nasty and unpleasant happened to you when you accidently fell off a cliff, or worse, if you were pushed. Standing under black roiling rainclouds got you wet from falling raindrops. You observed that these events only happened one way. Folks did not float up mysteriously from cliff bottoms, nor waters droplets rush up into the clouds from a lake. Rocks thrown at the nasty neighbors trying to steal your wife always fell back to earth if they didn't clonk the raiding party first.

Time was reckoned with the coming of each brand new day when the sun rose, then ending as the sun set, and the moon rose to light up his silvery night and bring on party time. Occasionally, when stuck deep inside his dark cave away from the sun, our caveman felt he somehow "knew" that a day was passing outside. Our caveman had not learned of daily circadian rhythms, or the brain's internal clock located in the suprachiasmic nucleus. The seasons rolled through a longer annual cycle, with game being scarce in the winter causing the growling of empty stomachs, and food abundant in the fat of summer as our caveman's prey brought forth their young. Birth and death in the human family marked out the limits and finality of human time.

Eventually, Newton came along and sorted out the spheres in the heavens, using his mathematical and mechanical genius to predict the transit of the planets across earth's skies with clockwork precision. As the poet and writer, Rudyard Kipling, would have put it: "God's in his heaven and all's right with the world." Then this little railway clerk, managing train timetables, came along and rocked Kipling's settled world and rattled our caveman brains. Einstein was able to cop a free ride or two on his trains to break the monotony of his boring job, and was fascinated by being on one train and watching a second train whizz by in the opposite direction on an adjoining rail track. Einstein, being something of a bright spark, was able to figure out that if each train was travelling at, say, 50 miles per hour, then their combined speed when hurtling past each other was 100 miles per hour.

Like most young men, when he wasn't chasing pretty young girls, Einstein was interested in power and speed. As in his time Einstein suffered from severe, total and absolute TIV deprivation syndrome (no TV, no Internet, no video games), he took to playing his own video games in his head. "What if I could cadge a ride on a light beam barreling through space at the max—700 *million* miles per hour?" Einstein thought. "That would be *sooo* cool, what a trip!" or whatever Swiss-German idiom of his time would express his youthful zest and enthusiasm.

Then, remembering his joy of being on a powerful train flying past another coming down the opposite track, Einstein cranked up his imagination another notch. He thought curiously, "What if I'm sitting on one light beam running at the max of 700 million miles per hour, the universe's speed limit, the speed of light, and another beam comes heading my way from the opposite direction, also hurtling at me at the maximum 700 million miles per hour?" That thought crossed his mind as he quickly grasped that the combined speed would be 1,400 million miles per hour!

Some stunt, he thought, then suddenly stopped. It was *verboten*, or forbidden, in his Swiss German, to exceed the universe's 700 million mile per hour speed limit. Einstein sat down and did his sums, then all hell broke loose. Our caveman concept of time was irrevocably shattered forever. Relativity theory was born, some say with the help of his wife, and time was merged with space and gravity.

On either side of the human scale, from the submicroscopic all the way up to the larger cosmos, time was relative, not absolute. It could go forward and backwards at the subatomic level, being essentially meaningless in comparison with our ancestral human terms. In the cosmos it merged with space and was warped by gravity. Einstein made light of his discovery and joked:

"The only reason for time is so that everything doesn't happen at once."
—Albert Einstein

The time that humankind had enjoyed for an eternity over the eons, as relayed by our poets, was severely challenged and essentially overthrown.

"Time and hour run through our roughest day."
—Shakespeare

Einstein, under his own challenges, reverted to the defensive when arguing his relativity theory, stubbornly pointing out that new discoveries always were scoffed and mocked by established science.

"If at first the idea is not absurd, then there is no hope for it."
—Albert Einstein

Einstein's incredible intellectual achievement, with his unification of time and space in his theories of relativity, opened a door into our way of thinking that will forever let in a breeze of incredulity.

"Reality is just an illusion, although a very persistent one."
—Albert Einstein

Our orderly worldview of time and space was subjected to a total revision, its implications startling, prompting the emergence of whole colleges of physicists attempting to unravel the novel and nuanced inferences. Explanations of how this impacts your self-help books' claims of directing your own future will draw on some of the newer theories of time. Additional perspective has been added to this quandary.

"No problem can be solved from the
same level of consciousness that created it."
—Albert Einstein

Imagine you are attempting to cross a fast-flowing stream. Whilst standing on the riverbank it is difficult to determine where the fordable shallows are and where the deep and dangerous currents run. At the eye level of the river's edge, your view and ability to analyze the situation is constrained and limited. You are frustrated by your lack of progress in choosing the right path and moving forward.

Now suppose you get the bright idea to climb a tall tree conveniently adjoining the river bank. With a few barked knuckles and scraped shins, you clamber up your tree. Immediately, you have literally moved into a new, vertical dimension. Your perspective is irreversibly transformed, with new relevant facts and information that you can use to understand the situation and its problems, and help plan a map towards your goal: getting safely to the other riverbank.

Now you can see the underlying flat rocks and sandbars that allow you to safely ford the stream. Your understanding of the various depths of the riverbed bottom has improved to the point where you can avoid the danger zones in your crossing. Introducing another new dimension has helped you grasp the underlying reality with greater perspicacity. Thinking differently, as Einstein advocated, helped solved your problem.

> *"We can't solve problems by using the same type of thinking that created them."*
> —Albert Einstein

The sandbox in which I played early on in my career was that of microscopy: electron, light and occasionally X-ray. We used these sophisticated microscopes to learn more as we visualized the biological scale from the size of the cell down to the molecular level. The energy used through the microscope lenses to image details of cells, mitochondria and viruses was to be found in the old familiar electromagnetic spectrum. Electron beams and light waves were the tools available. My thinking readily embraced the electromagnetic spectrum as the chief actor in the functioning of consciousness, in considering the workings of our brains.

When confronted with the challenge of explaining the seeming transmission between human minds, as in my dream with my father in pain six thousand miles distant, my thinking process was naturally boxed in from my work history, with my focus limited to the electromagnetic spectrum as the agency in play. *Mea culpa*, my timid explorations were all inside this box.

This left me with the challenge of explaining how sufficient levels of electromagnetic energy could be generated by a human brain to send so much data so far away. Also, what was the nature of the amplification process in the recipient brain—mine, on the receiving end of the dream? The death knell to this avenue of explanation was the Russian and American Faraday Cage screening experiments on gifted seers. Electromagnetic energy was effectively eliminated by the Faraday Cage screens around the seers, yet they could still "see" and call the pictographs on cards turned many yards away, above and beyond that predicted by statistical chance.

These paranormal seers' gifts did not require electromagnetism to function. Something else was allowing the transmission of data. Or, as the scientific authorities claimed, the statistics were weak, so the results were bogus, and my own mental forays into understanding my transformative dream were a futile waste of time and energy. Embarrassing and frustrating as this was to a former scientist, the power and veracity of my dream left my hopes untarnished. Back to the drawing board!

> *"If we knew what it was we were doing,*
> *it would not be called research, would it?"*
> —Albert Einstein

Quantum physics provided something of a lifeline, with particles popping in and out of existence in empty space. This represented a promising avenue for exploration of thought transmission. Amongst its many quirks, or quarks as the case may be, quantum physics has hard, repeatable, demonstrable experimental evidence of transmittal of information across vast distances.

Einstein himself had little patience for those who dabbled in parapsychology; however, he did believe, after a lifetime of work, as does Stephen Hawking (the discoverer of black holes that lie at the center of galaxies), that our universe and its underlying physics are explicable, and ultimately understandable (to at least *some* human minds). Observed events, even those seemingly paranormal at our present level of understanding, should thus be eventually comprehensible in physical terms. Quantum physics nudged my thinking outside the box, recognizing that it represented different dimensions, allowing an approach at a higher level than the lowly electromagnetic spectrum.

This book's purpose is an exploration of how your self-help books work. So, the hints, suggestions and occasional blatant declaration of thought projection into the future as a means to improve your life's story have a paranormal aspect that cannot be ignored. Moreover, as discussed above, objective events that occur in our lives deserve a scientific explanation even if they seem paranormal, and we do not as of yet have the science to understand and explain them. If the science is there, paranormality disappears.

A clear cut example of a prior "paranormal" experience being ushered under the umbrella of scientific rectitude popped up whilst I researched for this chapter on the internet. Couples with a long-standing relationship often experience the "sixth sense" of being tuned in uncannily to their mate's thoughts. Recently this happened to me; at the Sunday movies during the previews I turned to my spouse to raise and discuss a novel topic unrelated to the movie. Her response was the startling "I was just about to say the same thing to you."

Current studies by Australian researchers have clearly demonstrated that couples interacting in the laboratory develop synchronous brain waves and elicit the same thoughts. So what was once scoffed as "paranormal" now is availed the respectability of being subject to repeatable scientific scrutiny with appropriate instrumentation, to study brain waves that represent thoughts. These small revolutionary advances have not been lost on the parapsychology community, whose passionate beliefs in psychic phenomena are mostly dwarfed by the resounding lack of scientific theory and hard evidence. But they still may be right, awaiting science to catch up with their observations of abnormalities.

So many parapsychologists, hungry for answers like the rest of us and craving respectability, have just about fallen in love with quantum physics. Ridicule and scorn is poured on this "psi" crowd by many of the quantum physicists, with their lightning-fast crackerjack logic and greater in-depth knowledge of the field. A certain arrogant disdain seems inevitable, as the brainiacs fob off the weak intellectual meanderings of the psi workers reminiscent of the Biblical admonition:

"Cast ye not pearls before swine."
—Jesus Christ

Apparently even Jesus Christ had a tetchy way with words when the mood was upon him.

Unfortunately, the field of quantum physics leaves itself wide open to all sorts of abuse and misinterpretation. It is riddled with inherent unknowns, incomplete and conflicting theories, mathematics that is only available to those of high IQ and a working knowledge of its equations and values, and few physicists who can cross over into the biological field of neuroscience and consciousness, itself rife with mystery and incomprehension.

Most workers in the psi group honestly believe they have witnessed paranormal phenomena, and cling to the belief that parapsychology will help unravel the secrets of the universe, melding human consciousness with time, space and gravity in the tradition of the eastern mystics. Most of us would just be happy with tomorrow's winning lotto numbers.

Parapsychologists have glommed onto quantum physics as a path toward vindication, and to salve their own curiosity. The murky obscurity of the field aids and abets their pursuit, as even the most articulate physicists have their books trashed as "impenetrably dense" by book reviewers.

"Imaginary time is indistinguishable from direction in space."
—Stephen Hawking

Time has become a poster child for parapsychologists seeking to explain telepathy (thought reading across a distance) and seers who claim abilities to peek into the future on a frequent basis. This time conundrum was encapsulated by the mathematician and writer, Lewis Carroll, when he had the Red Queen in *Alice in Wonderland* declare to Alice: "It's a poor memory that only works backwards."

The psychologist Carl Jung spent a large part of his career evolving his thoughts on coincidences that occur in our lives. Jung engaged the quantum physicist, Wolfgang Pauli, in this pursuit, and coined the term "synchronicity" to describe the coincidences we all experience, and are sometimes used by self-help books as evidence for laws of attraction.

To Jung, synchronicity meant much more than mere coincidence. He felt it reflected a revelation of a deeper structure to our world, demonstrating a meaningful unifying connection between our human time experience and the real outer world. He may well have been right. However, although he was a highly intelligent man who sought and recruited some of the best brains on quantum physics in his generation, Jung was never able to advance his claim, nor develop and articulate his synchronicity theme much beyond establishing its existence.

However, we have all felt it: that strange uncanny experience with our thoughts ranging on an old friend, or nondescript topic, only out of the blue suddenly to have it pop up into our lives. The reader will no doubt have numerous examples of his own with which to identify. Your self-help books often seize upon this coincidence as proof of their veracity and trustworthiness. I recount a simple personal instance of synchronicity that occurred to me with relevance to the writing of this book as an example below.

One of my pleasures in life, after my evening workout, is to loll on my couch in my study under my reading lamp with a stack of books at hand, and occasionally I relax my eyes by raising my gaze to enjoy watching the ocean breezes caress the leaves on the trees outside my window.

Recently, whilst enjoying the novel *God is an Englishman* by R. F. Delderfield, I put it down to muse on the value to this chapter of incorporating different dimensions as possible explanations of self-help book claims into this chapter. I focused on time, as the future is of prime interest in self-help development.

My books on quantum consciousness were readily at hand in my stack, and I rooted through them and pored over some salient points on the physics of time and took some notes. Then, without further ado, I resumed reading my novel about the travails of its semi-comatose hero. Imagine how I felt when turning the page the very next sentence to hit my eye read: "Time was the element that eluded him." I felt a little tingle run through me. Synchronicity at play, stunningly explicit, whatever its explanation.

The study of time and how this reflects on your self-help books' manifestations is wrought with the pitfalls of our limited under-standing of Einstein's melding of time into space. For example, the end of time exists already in our universe. How bizarre is that to the caveman mind? Within those objects of pure gravity, black holes, Hawking assures us that time ceases to exist.

"Anything that falls through the event horizon will reach a region of infinite density and the end of time *"*
—Stephen Hawking

One reason time importantly affects self-help efforts is the apparent willing of future events through control of our human consciousness. Some physicists make the startling conclusion that time exists in chunks, or loops. These time loops can and do embrace present, past and future relative to our human plane of existence. Should the reader happen to find himself inside one of these time loops, he could experience a seeming miraculous encounter with the future. So if this be true, can our focused thoughts elicit such events more frequently with increased encroachment into time loops, than if we just mindlessly went about our day-to-day business? When and if the physicists can get their stories straight on this one, it opens fresh fields for the neurophysiologists to prove that our minds do indeed have these apparent miraculous powers.

At its basic level, self-help claims that new helpful thoughts, future presciences, events or opportunities are jumping up into our lives, whereas without our focused thought, we are stuck with the bland banality of random chance. This is reminiscent of Einstein's "spooky effects at a distance" which he admitted he could not account for.

"The intellect has little to do on the road to discovery.
There comes a leap in consciousness, call it intuition or what you will,
the solution comes to you and you don't know how or why."
—Albert Einstein

However, Einstein's own relativity theories led to the understanding that in reality, past, present and future all occur at the same time, at least at the quantum level of the subatomic particle. Change is the only reality in relativity. Some physicists claim the existence of subatomic particles that are discrete units of time, hypothetical tachyons (that can move faster than the speed of light), whilst other physicists deride this notion, stating that there are no infinitely small demonstrable divisible units of time, which can only thus exist as a flow.

The debate rages on, leaving the caveman brain gasping for air.

We readily acknowledge recognizable change in our aphorisms for the changes we observe in the human lifespan. The old adage encapsulates this with a touch of bittersweet irony: A woman marries a man hoping to change him, whereas a man marries a woman hoping she never changes.

Such is the stuff of humanity.

Changes brought about by the stepwise inverse Zeno induction process reviewed earlier, also known as backward causal changes or causal time loops, may disappear and cease to exist if one enters into the mathematics of many dimensions or multidimensional space. The introduction of multidimensional space into the scenario alters the basic properties of these steps or chunks of time, permitting them to all cohabit and exist together at the same moments in time.

Progression forward or backward, one from the other, is therefore irrelevant in this mathematical world of small multiple dimensions. Some self-help books sanction these effects to extend up from the submicroscopic to our human size scale. The books then state this categorically as a truth, arguing that if everything already exists, then it's just a matter of your lining up your conscious thoughts to select your desired pre-existing or co-existing desired condition from this cornucopia. Your obligation is thus to develop enough emotional steam or vigor to manifest the selected goal from this panoply of choices. Heady stuff indeed!

What is important in this approach to time is that better knowledge of where the physicists are taking us could help illuminate some of the wilder, almost magical effects promoted in the self-help literature. Physicists themselves claim that if we understood the nature of time properly in these other invisible dimensions, then the apparent jumps or inconsistencies of particles, thoughts and events just reflect a human blindness to their presence all around us, all the time. Explicable and logically consistent in the mathematics of the physicists, but magic to our caveman brains.

If you thought you were done with this time stuff, please bear with me, as there is more to come. The next step in grasping how thoughts and events can miraculously pop up out of nowhere by virtue of your thoughts is to accept the physicists' claim that all things are there all the time in other dimensions and, yes, other universes. It's only "nowhere" to our human senses. We just need to drop our inadequately evolved blinkers.

Physicists have grown enough horse sense for them to understand that the use of multiple dimension theories and multiple universes, where many different outcomes for your life run in parallel, probably reflect an even deeper level of understanding than we now possess or can articulate with our earthbound evolution of language. Let me lighten up a little on you now, with a bit of biology.

Intriguingly, many of the writers and proponents of the eight, ten, eleven or twenty-six dimensions are female physicists. Females apparently have more curiosity about hidden dimensions. Traditionally, physicists have been male, the necessary mathematical trait believed to be enhanced by am overabundant flood of testosterone from the developing fetal testes, impacting the fetal brain during the first and second trimester before birth.

The focus on mathematics in the male may border on autism, with its limited social abilities. Sir Isaac Newton himself is now considered to have been autistic and somewhat of a social cripple. As mathematicians also have to earn a living, Newton did a stint as Master of His Majesty's Royal Mint. In this role he policed the integrity of the coinage, and showed callous disregard for those who would clip gold from the edges of his sovereign's coin of the realm, or forge its currency. Newton frequently ordered that such criminals suffer execution by the gory English standards of those days. He had them hung, disemboweled, or "drawn," then butchered into four pieces.

So, using the technology of advanced mathematics to explore additional dimensions, the inconsistent jumps of events found repeatedly in experimental physics for the very small subatomic particles, and the larger human-size manifestations predicted in your self-help books, are all just part of larger pre-existing consistent continuum when extra dimensions are invoked. Arthur C. Clarke's observation that a "sufficiently advanced technology can be indistinguishable from magic" is obviously applicable to this situation, and could not ring more true.

Our earlier analogy of climbing a tree to obtain a better perspective to successfully ford a river, by moving into another dimension, is certainly applicable to our better understanding of apparent jumps in time, when multiple dimensions are brought into play. These will only be understood, if ever, by adhering to Einstein's simple but eloquent admonition that problems must be solved using a higher type of thinking than those that created them.

Below the subatomic level, where quantum mechanics rules the roost, physicists continue their brilliant forays into the unknown. Vibrational packages of energy, known as "strings" in string theory, are thought to be the next level down in our hierarchical way of thinking, as the underlying constituent matter of subatomic particles. Until recently, the existence of strings, and hence string theory itself, has had little if any experimental evidence to back it up and substantiate its validity in the hard concrete terms demanded and respected by science.

Small advances continue to trickle out of the theoretical physicists and may point the way to firming up string theory. The pure gravity of our universe's black holes may be "leaking" in an osmotic fashion back out into the universe through the plane or screen of the event horizon. Some believe that this may represent the stuff we call "dark energy" that is responsible for the observed expansion of the universe.

If this proves to be true, some physicists believe that it will provide them an experimental platform to test the math of string theory. Its arcane esoterica is beyond this book's scope, but suffice to say it involves marrying strings to quantum behavior known as entanglement. How this will redound to new understanding of human consciousness is a way down the pike, but the cross-fertilization between physics and neurobiology will continue unabated.

So, what if anything lies below the level of the vibrating strings? What entities make up the very infinitesimal and final reality that constitutes the matter of which we and the universe are all made? How will this new knowledge impact future revisions of this book and our understanding of our minds? Some theorists posit "pure information" without expounding on its makeup.

However, they don't just grab these ideas out of a hat after a night on the ale (or maybe they do), and in order to withstand the critiques of their formidable peers, they are obligated to back up their suggestions with models to prove or disprove them. The "information is the very very bottom element" group advocate a model whereby the black hole event horizon is a holographic screen of pure information. This model will permit analysis for verification or dismissal of "information" as the final arbiter of the essence of the universe.

This sketch of additional types of thinking or levels of thought is shared with you to provide a glimpse of mankind's incredible intellectual achievements thus far, even with the caveman brain, and how it may impinge on deciphering self-help. Meanwhile, we all still have to live in our real world of familiar human time, as when last orders are called, and the publican drapes his bar towel across his beer pumps and intones "Time, gentlemen please."

CHAPTER ELEVEN

RESONANCE, ATTRACTION AND PROVIDENCE

"Until one is committed there is hesitancy, the chance to draw back, always ineffectiveness. Concerning all acts of initiative and creation there is one elementary truth, the ignorance of which kills countless ideas and splendid plans: that moment one definitely commits oneself then PROVIDENCE moves too. All sorts of things occur to help one that never would otherwise occurred.

A whole stream of events issues from that decision, raising in one's favor all manner of unforeseen incidents and meetings and material assistance, which no man could have dreamt would have come his way.

I have learned a deep respect for one of Goethe's couplets:
'Whatever you can do, or dream you can, begin it.
Boldness has a power and magic in it.'"
—William Hutchinson Murray, Scottish mountain climber

It goes by many names in your self-help books, but it is always there, always featured prominently, and with good reason. It works. You are not being steered wrong; however, the spicy, tarted-up language may be misleading or easily misunderstood.

Providence, servo-mechanism, goal fulfillment mechanism, 'law 'of attraction and the rest, can alternate in meaning from some quasi-magical external force to the inner workings of our brains, as the agency that brings about your wish gratification.

The providence in Murray's writings was due in his mind to the commitment he had made in cold hard cash. Although Liverpool born, Murray was raised in Scotland and knew the value of hard-earned money. He committed himself to climbing Mount Everest the moment he put down his passage money, booking a sailing to Bombay, India. Events took off from there, and although hampered by altitude sickness was able to join in the Scottish Himalayan expedition to Everest.

Murray's mysticism was cemented into his mind during an earlier wartime experience during the battle of El Alamein against the German tank commander, Field Marshall Rommel. This battle, the first victory the British had against the Nazis that helped turn the tide in World War Two, resulted in Murray's capture and horrific experiences in German hands as a prisoner of war. Prior to his capture, Murray underwent a life-changing psychic experience that helped sustain him during the miseries and suffering of his prison camps.

During sustained shelling which cut Murray's dispatch runner in half at the waist, yet left him running toward him "smoking at the waist" in Murray's words, another shell created a bomb crater right next to Murray. Received wisdom of the troops was that shells never fell in the same place twice, and offered a modicum of shelter from the next barrage.

Yet just as Murray was about to crawl for protection into the crater, an external voice filled his entire mind. "STOP! Don't move!" It shook Murray to the core, this overwhelming command blocking out all other thought, vividly and powerfully demanding he stay still, away from the newly created bomb crater. Sure enough, the very next shell that came sailing through the air towards him landed in the exact same crater against all odds and exploded, whence he would surely had had his life instantly snuffed out were he in it.

Obviously Murray thought this over many times to characterize each life-saving minutiae of this explosive mental entreaty, during the long hours and years of his captivity. He recalls the intensity of that commanding voice was entirely absolute in its demand, brooking no dissent, clearly emanating from outside himself, yet flooding his brain overcoming any conscious logical thought. And no, there were no other soldiers in his vicinity: this was a nonhuman command. Whilst in the camps he had time to meditate and mingle with others who shared mystical beliefs, but Murray adamantly maintained that this was his one and only psychic experience, and never enjoyed another throughout his long life.

This experience was certainly providential, but fails to meet the steady goal seeking timeframe of attraction laws of your self-help books, nor is it explicable in terms of today's physics. Something real and life-saving happened to William Murray that day, instantaneously and beyond anything this book, or any courageous physicist can currently explain.

Just how the forces unleashed by your self-help efforts are able to manifest your desired results is never fully explained in your self-help books, except in vague, unsatisfactory metaphysical terms. Some propose a resonance or harmonic vibration of your thoughts with like-minded objects out there in the universe or multiverse. This represents a challenge for those of who relish a more complete understanding of how our chosen wishes transmute into hard, physical, tangible objects like a one-hundred-dollar bill. Because all of us have at some point in our lives experienced this attraction, and although it can appear almost miraculously uncanny, no satisfactory underlying mechanism is discussed in the self-help books.

Our brains do, however, have a well-known and well-studied built-in system that may fit the bill. This system involves arousal or mental stimulation. It is located at the top half of our brain stem, where automatic functions are regulated, and the lower part of the cerebral cortex where mental calculation and input can occur. This is internal, part of our brain inside our heads, not out there somewhere in the universe. Its function does not require or rely upon some unknown, unstudied and uncharacterized resonance with the universe. It can alert us to our needs by overriding our built-in mental filters, creating spurts of arousal, when we spy our wants in our vicinity. It is called the Reticular Activating System, or RAS.

This book has gotten to this chapter deliberately without naming names in the self-help community in an attempt to maintain a respectable impartiality. It also allows whatever scientific evidence that can be scraped together in support and substantiation to be presented to you, the reader, in order that you can form your own judgment and reach your own thoughtful conclusions. The exception proves the rule, and in this instance the thoughts and writings on our "servo-mechanism" as put forward by the plastic surgeon and author Dr. Maxwell Maltz in his books on "Psychocybernetics" forms a close approximation to the workings of the RAS.

Oftentimes when we focus on, say, buying a particular car, it seems to crop up whenever we are on the road, ostensibly every-where we look, with regularity and an almost eerie predictability, whereas our choice automobile barely registered prior to our thoughts on acquiring it. How can this be if we don't believe in magic? Our sage, Arthur C. Clarke, is again apropos, with his observation we have used repeatedly and appropriately before in this book: "sufficiently advanced technology can appear to be magic." What if the sufficiently advanced technology is already hardwired into our brains, and how does it work?

Our brain acts as a filter. We would quickly go mad, rapidly sliding into insanity in minutes, if we perceived every input our senses can detect in our surrounding environment. The sights, smells, tastes, sounds and tactile sensations of our closely approximate world we all come into contact with second by second would flood and overwhelm our consciousness with such an overload of data that life would be unbearable. Is it coincidental that the part of the electromagnetic spectrum—visible light, to which about one third of our brain is used to process—only occupies about one-billionth of the entire electromagnetic spectrum? Our brains can only handle so much input.

Evolution has provided us with mental filters to screen out the unimportant, and less important, in the data stream that inundates us. If it doesn't directly affect our survival it waits in line, or is just filtered out and ignored. This helps dampen down our arousal mechanisms so that we are not constantly on guard for danger, and can enjoy a measure of serenity and tranquility.

We have all had days with information overload or TMI—Too Much Information—especially in these times of the internet, tweets and instant messaging making us a little confused, cross and irritable. All mankind seeks occasional solace on a quiet (low input) beach, lake or woodland glade, even if only in our imagination. Authors of novels spend whole paragraphs painting mental pictures of such environments, creating an atmospheric scene in which their protagonists play out their given roles.

When you want to jack up your senses and actually increase the enjoyable thoughts concerning a vitally desired goal, those new shoes or handbag you've just got to have, or that dream car you want so much in your driveway, then you begin to see the wanted object more frequently, seemingly everywhere, your car on the highways, your shoes on someone else with that matching designer bag. What is happening to you to make this happen? Is this some immutable 'law' of attraction that your focused positive thoughts have energized somehow the universe to fulfill the old adage: What you want, wants you?

Your subconscious got the message. The intense emotional focus that occupied most of your thought channels has been picked up and processed by your subconscious as something very important to the organism—you—it is operating within. Your subconscious primes your reticular activating system, or RAS, to unlock your mental filters and help scan your environment for clues and details that will bring you closer to your chosen goal. Your RAS responds to a hit or sighting of your intended new purchase with increased arousal, ensuring that you don't miss or filter out the signals from your environment that have been present all along, always there and ubiquitous, but previously and normally damped down and ignored.

The increased sightings can for all intents and purposes appear magical. You say "Aha! These self-help laws of attraction really work!" It is as if your very wanting, your deep and needy craving of a thing, brings it into reality in your life. Your thoughts resemble those of a poet's pen, bringing airy nothings into a concrete form.

"As imagination bodies forth, the form of things unknown,
the poets pen turns them into shape, and gives to airy nothing a
local habitation and a name, such tricks had strong imagination."
—Shakespeare

Unlike Shakespeare's recognition that it is the internal imagination that is transmuted into hard realty, the self-help books proclaim that some external force or entity is now aligned with your magnetism, thus manifesting those new designer shoes. However, it is just you and your brain, with its adjusted internal RAS scanner, picking up the bleeps of your intended purchase like a radar sweep.

So far the science holds, but is that all there is to it? Let me share a simple personal story, with another distinction or wrinkle to illustrate that other factors may be in play and your self-help books may actually have cottoned on to another underlying reality.

My old car was nearing the end of its lease and needed replacement. As I hail from the old country, I retain that Englishman's fascination of my generation with sports cars. True enough, once I got the idea in my head, and even visited the sports car showroom, I saw my intended sports car buzzing about on southern California's freeways and highways. My RAS was clicking along in high gear and functioning in the accepted manner discussed above.

The distinction, the little intriguing wrinkle, that may reveal another underlying aspect to this phenomenon, was my desire to examine the car more closely and talk to an owner of this relatively rare little beauty. I wanted the input of an owner to garner more details on handling, performance and the location of other dealerships to develop my pre-purchase research.

I couldn't get the damn car out of my mind as I pulled into a huge shopping warehouse lot to buy some electronics for my office. This was during pre-recession days and the parking lot was full to the brim. I just managed to squeeze into the last remaining slot, carefully walked around my car after locking it, and went into the store to select my purchase.

Returning to my car with my shopping bag, I was entranced to see that out of that entire parking full lot of hundreds of mundane cars, a space had opened up in front of mine. You guessed it: the car pulling in was the rare gem I was interested in. Not only that, it was a souped-up version with an enthusiastic owner overly eager to spend time with me chatting about its virtues. Just what I had been obsessing about.

So, my rational brain well understood that the sightings on the freeways were a direct result of my reprogrammed RAS, but this was at an entirely different level of involvement. This could not be explained by RAS enhancement alone. The low odds of all the particulars of the encounter coming together pointed to a more fundamental aspect, or deeper interaction of my passionate thoughts than mere chance alone.

Science expands and grows, often after encountering that niggling little anomaly that just doesn't fit in, or mesh with the current extant theory. The nagging inconsistency sometime points to another truth that we have been missing, overlooked by our ready acceptance of the prevailing explanations. From this, new experiments and understanding can incrementally blossom.

> *"People think of these eureka moments and my feeling is that they tend to be little things, a little realization, and then a little realization built on that."*
> —Roger Penrose, physicist

Could some quantum events such as the inverse Zeno phenomenon play a role in zeroing you in on your target? It is not ruled out. We as of yet just don't know enough how our universe works to explain it. Some physicists suggest that resonance between two systems (you and your desired car, for example) increase the amount of energy considerably. When two objects vibrate at the same frequency, or in phase, or exhibit resonance, then there is more energy to attract themselves to each other than if they were out of synchrony, or out of phase. If out of phase, lacking such resonance, two objects would more likely *repel* each other.

There are anecdotal reports of gamblers who play the lottery, *a priori* bragging to friends and family that they are going to win it and start spending money like drunken sailors in anticipation of their stupendous luck. Lo and behold, these braggarts actually win. Well, that's a one-off you might think, just a coincidence, a highly improbable coincidence, but a coincidence nevertheless, and just shrug it off. Then they do it again! A repetition of the first episode of braggadocio, with another lottery win. The odds of this happening are astronomical, unless they have a shill on the inside fixing the lottery results. One can be excused in the face of such anecdotes, such strange statistical anomalies, of hearing strains of the *Twilight Zone* whispering through your head, and feel the hairs stand up on the back of your neck.

However, the gist of this book is to move understanding forward, no matter how pitifully slowly, using whatever science we can muster, without recourse to new age mysticism. The reason being for this is that a lot of self-help books actually work, for very rational reasons. Granted, it's a mixed bag with spiritualistic mumbo-jumbo thrown in to hype sales, but some of the fundamentals remain strong and true.

> "*What we truly and earnestly aspire to be, that,* in some sense we are. *The mere aspiration, by changing the frame of mind,* for the moment realizes itself."
> —Anna Jameson, nineteenth-century writer

CHAPTER TWELVE

PUTTING YOUR THOUGHTS TO WORK IN YOUR LIFE

"God helps those who help themselves."
—Aesop's Greek Fables

No matter how wretched and depressing your current circumstances, find comfort in the fact that your self-help book does indeed offer you at least one key, honest, fundamental and truthful basic tenet. You may be suffering from "the slings and arrows of misfortune" as Shakespeare would have put it, but your self-help tomes offer you the way out.

You may currently be unfortunate to be living through a hell of any of the following: in jail doing time, a boringly stifling dead-end job, a souring personal relationship, pain and suffering of a long-term illness or the tyranny of a megalomaniacal boss or government, but your self-help book offers one piece of supreme and cardinal lifesaving and life-changing advice. It is this: you, and you alone, can become *aware* of your thoughts. You can then *change* your thoughts. This, however, is not something new to the human race.

"As the bowman makes straight his arrows,
so the wise man straightens his unsteady mind."
—Buddha, Dhammapada 300BC

Awareness and thought control are stressed in your self-help books as the first step on you road to self-improvement. This practice was developed and utilized earlier in the East. From it came a sense of understanding the universe that meshes with and closely resembles that proposed by our modern quantum physicists. Appreciation of this convergence or amalgamation of eastern mysticism and its challenging linguistics, with modern physics with its equally abstruse language, has led some of the new age persuasion to go a little overboard.

Melding all into one has encouraged some to go all gaga over Buddhist philosophy. There has been an overreach based on this adoption of ersatz Buddhism which rings a little phony and smacks of wish fulfillment. For those of the commune conviction, with its fake kum-by-yah comradeship, this seeming scientific vindication of their adopted Buddhist philosophy is used as justification for an uncritical pollyannaism. So, what are the facts behind this philosophy, and how might they bear on your self-help efforts?

You may be wondering how a guy named Buddha on the Indian subcontinent around twenty-five hundred years ago got around to thinking through the very essence of the universe, which some say is on a par with modern physics. What's more, how did such a technologically unsophisticated wanderer come so close to the concepts discovered by the European scientists with all their instruments as they unraveled the secrets and mysteries of quantum physics on which modern self-help heavily rests, in the nineteenth and twentieth centuries? Enquiring minds want to know: who was this guy Buddha?

A spoilt little rich kid, born in Nepal in 560 BC, Buddha was a prince. His dad, the king, wanted young Buddha to follow in his footsteps and become the next monarch. The king did not want his son to enter the priesthood of his time, and become an ascetic monk as predicted by the court's royal astrologers, and exercised all his royal might to prevent this from happening.

Dad therefore kept his son, Buddha, in a gilded cage. No expense was spared as the young man grew up ensconced in a walled estate, a pleasure garden filled with fountains, beautiful women and music, shielded from the poverty, sickness, squalor and decrepitude that was 545 BC Nepal. Buddha married one of his consorts at age sixteen and enjoyed a totally privileged life away from the surrounding poverty of the Nepalese masses.

Curiosity, and the urge to wander and explore, overcame the young prince. After being sheltered from the human condition with its ravages of age, poverty, disease and death all his impressionable young life, Buddha's witnessing of these miseries in the city streets outside his pleasure garden's walls had a profound transformative effect on his young mind.

The shock of witnessing mortality and morbidity of other human beings in disease-wracked bodies, so unlike the lissome creatures he was used to, was ameliorated when Buddha met a calm, mellow understanding monk. So impressed and infatuated was the callow Buddha by the monk's serene acceptance of mankind's lot, that Buddha renounced his life of luxury and comfort (no word of what happened to the wife) to take up the monastic life with the words:

"World happiness is transitory."
—Buddha

After a stint of severe training in abstention, whence Buddha almost starved to death, and meditation and yoga breathing exercises which had been learned and practiced long before Buddha's arrival on planet earth by cave-dwelling hermits in the Nepalese foothills, Buddha was able to meditate deeply on his own. Following one particular prolonged meditation, Buddha emerged and announced that he had experienced a revelatory trance whereby he had achieved the state of nirvana.

Describing this state of nirvana to the western mind challenges even the 750,000 words available in the English language. Nirvana reflects a sought-after goal of meditators where all anguish and delusion is extinguished from your thoughts and a state of bliss, with an all-knowing knowledge, is enjoyed.

Similar all-knowing knowledge is forecast by some astrophysicists in our times. Our widely held concept of our universe expanding at incredible rates from the singular point or singularity of the Big Bang has been book- ended by some physicists to be balanced by a "Big Crunch" singularity, or omega point, at the end of our universe.

The key comparison to nirvana is that as our universe violently contracts, shearing the very stuff of atoms to smithereens, vast amounts of energy are released which in turn accelerate computational ability speeds with logarithmic rises of intensity. Knowledge balloons so rapidly as to be all-encompassing, as in nirvana, that whosoever has this nirvana-knowledge can escape their rapidly impending doom, even within microseconds of the final omega collapse. Their overwhelming nirvana-knowledge allows them to escape into any unlimited virtual reality worlds of their own thoughts and choosing, selecting, manifesting and living in their own newly created heavens. Now that's thinking!

Back to Buddha: after his transformative epiphany and dance with nirvana, he continued to obsess over his nirvana of joy with more meditations and writings on his observations of the human condition. Buddha's sense of oneness with the universe, achieved in the nirvana state, convinced him he could and did experience all the knowledge and truth of the universe in these meditations, whereby he renounced all need for normal human desires.

The arcane language of his esoteric sense of immersion and dissociative loss of self (which we associate with psychotic states) in a seemingly all-encompassing sense of pure being is hard to translate into modern terms. Those who have experienced the chemical imbalance of their brains with LSD hallucinogenic trips claim to have enjoyed similar dissociative, out of this world rapture, described by Aldous Huxley as "opening the doors of perception" with a powerful sense of God-like omniscience. The inventor of the iPod, Steve Jobs, described his LSD experiences as "one of the two or three most important things he had done in his life."

Buddha's undoubted wisdom was transcribed into sacred writings for centuries after his death, in much the same way the Bible's New Testament was written, copied, confabulated and re-written after Christ's death. Another moral reformer, Confucius, born in China in 479 BC after Buddha's death, was so sickened by the corruption around him that he latched onto and expanded Buddhist precepts, which in turn were again expanded, added to and developed by his contemporary, Lao Tse (or Tzu, meaning mature wise old man). Thus the eastern mysticism of Tao Buddhism was developed.

This melding of moral strictures on how to live, with the profound insights as to the natures of thought, consciousness, matter and the universe, came down to us in the western world under the generic umbrella term Buddhism. It must be remembered that much of this philosophy and meditative practice preceded Buddha's actual life. Buddha inherited his meditative skills from the nameless Nepalese hermits who had long practiced these arts in the Himalayan foothills in the ages before him.

They inherited this knowledge from the basis of the Hindu religion, the Rig Veda, a series of 1,028 poems and hymns, derived from Aryan invaders from Siberia who settled in northwest India and written in 1700-1100 BC. Over one-tenth of these insightful verses were written under the influence of a brown drink "soma," made from stalks of *Ephedra sinica*, whose drug use was rejoiced in these same verses.

> *"We have gone to the light, and found the gods."*
> —Veda poem

The psychoactive drug is ephedrine, which gave a speed- or ecstasy-type high. Whether or not Buddha took this form of ecstasy before his insightful meditations is unknown.

The concept of nirvana, permanent enlightened understanding, was undoubtedly taught to Buddha by the monks who took him under their wing, as a welcome escape after the shock of seeing death and disease ravage the poor folks. The monks' superstructure embodied all the moral strictures of abstention, chastity, long-standing traditions of asceticism, use of plant euphorics, and of course, meditative yoga breathing practices as the quickest trip to nirvana.

In order for us to find our way back to our caves and around the rocks strewn in our path, our brains have evolved a neat little apparatus at the back of the head in the posterior subparietal nucleus, with the grand name of the Orientation Association Center, or OAA. Its job is to stay alert and guide us through obstacles in a room, by letting you know where your body is in time and space. Accident victims whose OAA is damaged have a real difficulty of knowing where there body is in space, hence trouble in moving around.

Interestingly, when experienced Buddhist monks meditate under appropriate brain scanning, when they are approaching the sense of oneness with the universe with loss of the normal sharp distinction between self and non-self (the OAA's job), blurring the line between feeling "in body" and "out of body," the OAA is seen to shut down and become quiescent or asleep. So, this state of nirvana, once believed of the paranormal realm, may be in part due to natural, if abnormal, self-induced brain changes.

As Tao Buddhism migrated into Japan, another word, satori, pops up in the eastern literature. Satori, unlike long-lasting nirvana, appears closer to our word epiphany, in that it is of a more transitory nature than the impactful nirvana state with its long duration. We in the West would consider it closer to the Pauline transformation of the formerly sour, cantankerous Saul to the newly enlightened and love-filled Paul on his trek along the road to Damascus. Satori would equate to a flash of insight.

Zealots of the Buddhist persuasion, whilst acknowledging the profoundly moral and perceptive teachings of Buddha's revelations, can occasionally lapse into a smug conceit, capriciously bandying about these words that are foreign to our ears. The assumption is a definitely non-Buddhist sense of smug self-satisfied superiority, coupled with a mind-numbing lack of clarity and obfuscation as to their own lack of comprehension, whilst at the same time retaining the pride and esteem of belonging to an exclusive in-group.

The reality is that these proponents—Buddha, Confucius and Lao Tse—were all real living people, not gods. They learned and grew as they went along, experiencing the harsh realities of their times. Yet they were able to develop and record in their primitive world their erudite visions of a pure consciousness permeating man and the universe. This pure consciousness, which in our times is a bedrock of self-help access to your future events, is variously described as a unified field, field of energy, or ocean of pure consciousness, adopted by the quantum physicists to explain their experiments, and ultimately the omega point end of time. No mean feat for the Buddhists!

Yet in the interest of fairness to latter-day western Buddhists, it may reflect the fact the Buddha's limited vocabulary itself, hampered the ability to communicate his thinking clearly, as his attempts to describe his nirvana painfully show:

"There is no meditation without wisdom, and there is no wisdom without meditation. When a man has both meditation and wisdom he is indeed close to nirvana."
—Buddha

Fast forward to the twentieth century, with the quantum physicist's assessment and definition, in a Swiss-German's English of a nirvana-like oneness with the universe, and our human denial of omniscient consciousness:

"A human being is part of the whole, called by us the universe,
a part limited in time and space. He experiences himself,
his thoughts and feeling as something separate from the rest—
a kind of optical delusion of his consciousness."
—Einstein

And you wonder why your self-help books have a hard time coming to grips with a sensible and understandably clear definition of universal consciousness or the universe's energy field? Nevertheless, it is this master mind or global subconscious that is purported by your self-help book to give you that leg up as you strive for goal achievement, as providence moves to assist you, when you tap into it with your newly focused thoughts. Does physics support this universal mind? That's the question.

Although it may seem like I am flogging a dead horse to crunch down onto a better-tasting definition of the poorly defined universal energy field, if you understand it to be true, the easier will come your faith and ultimate trust in your self-help's guide to your progress. An old nineteenth-century idea posited that light was transmitted through an all-surrounding "aether" which pervaded all matter, including us. Light studies showed this was equivocally not so, there was no "aether." But the concept is close to the universal human supraconsciousness of all humanity, equating to an all-pervading energy field, and lingers on in the self-help literature without hard proof or evidence.

The particles (thoughts?) that pop in and out of existence, and so much loved by those attempting to extrapolate quantum physics to human mental machinations (such as explored in this book), can be considered not as new, *de novo* apparitions, but being there all the time, albeit in different form. The proposed field that surrounds us contains ephemeral, nebulous waves awaiting their day in the sun through the act of observation, whence their wave form instantaneously collapses into a discrete, concrete identifiable particle. Voila! Now you see it, now you don't, something from nothing—it's magic!

"No sweat," you say, "I've got this pregnant energy field down pat by now, only it doesn't take nine months to manifest a new birth, it's instantaneous." Next question. Observation? Hmmm, what's that? And who is the observer? Physicists scrupulously avoid defining observer and observation when it comes to such manifestations. "Well, it's my thought, just like my self-help book taught me, that acts as observer and makes the act of observation," you may say. And, against all logic and proof, this does appear to be one case, validating your self-help book, but again awaiting further advances in physics and the English vocabulary to create language and depth of understanding of the observation enigma. "Observation" will no doubt be replaced with different language at that future unfolding.

Most readers with an open mind probably adhere to an atheistic or, when pushed, an agnostic bent, skirting the issue of God as the observer for all those events that pop into existence that we don't have time to think about. Without impugning those of a religious calling, it does seem something of a cop-out, a failure in our science to discern underlying truths that keep our whole playground floating through the sky.

In contrast to German's 300,000 words, our English language boasts over 750,000. Yet this remains insufficient to describe adequately and get to the gist of a marriage between the riddles of eastern mysticism and the mysteries revealed in the quantum world. That is also a challenge of your self-help books, which attempt to dogmatically assert with authoritarian argument the existence of a supra-conscious universal all-knowing nirvana- type mind that is at one with the energy field of the universe. In the end, you just have to take it on faith, believe it's true and move on.

As you begin to train your thoughts in keeping with the instruction from your self-help book, with awareness and then direction of thought, you may discover other types of thinking than our traditional western goal-seeking fantasies. Samatha is a different method of using your mind, and is achieved in the Buddhist tradition to achieve an escapist, relaxing, abiding calm from daily stress. Samatha is achieved through deep controlled breathing meditation, in a yoga fashion, self-monitoring your breathing pattern, in an attempt at cooling off the mind to attain a state of mindful, sustained attention that can last for hours, whilst basking in the pacification of a serene, pristine tranquility.

Does the western mind have the capability to achieve a similar state without the discipline of self-monitored breathing meditation? After all, we have the same bodies and brains of our eastern colleagues. Our words would embrace and identify samatha with terms such as trance, fugue or reverie. Some westerners feel they can enter a cataleptic ecstasy listening to classical music. Others induce an abstracted stupor or somnambulism with injected or inhaled hypnotic chemicals. Monastic orders sing repetitive chants to attain a sense of grace, a saintly disembodied rapture.

Readers may have their own reminisces of this dream state as I recount a post-prandial episode on a close, muggy day, back in high school. Ensconced in a temporary postwar classroom, with the rain thrumming on the roof reflecting a typical English summer, my mind readily slipped in a beautiful, comfortable, relaxed, settled and thoughtless daydream. This quiet trance and blissful fugue state seemingly stretched into eternity as our English Lit teacher droned on and on.

It was a mental state I visited frequently in the high school classroom, and is common enough that most readers have probably also felt and enjoyed this tranquil escapist bliss. Typically, it was violently shattered by my little pugnacious English teacher bellowing out my name, utterly wasting my muse, destroying my enjoyable reverie. His demand that I expostulate to the class on the antics of one of Jane Austen's gold-digging heroines put paid to my cheap mental vacation.

So, yes, we humans across the centuries can experience similar mental states without resorting to meditation or yoga. But what prompted those overactive animated minds of the nineteenth century to delve into the mysteries of the quantum world? These scientists were not impoverished monks, glorifying in sensory deprivation and meditating in mountain caves in Nepal, but a bunch of relatively wealthy white guys with too much time on their hands and a nosy inquisitive bent. Nevertheless, their brilliant perceptiveness, so unlike the mush of our commonplace daydreams, added to their musings and intellectual insights, helped usher in the modern era.

One key difference to their predecessors in the East was the development of science. This tool had been honed though the centuries in the West, first developing a hypothesis, then testing it experimentally with apparatus in the laboratory to prove their thesis right or wrong. This went by the name of classical deterministic science, as they were able to determine truth through the verification of experimental observation of results.

As our womenfolk are constantly chiding us, men like to play with toys. The laboratories of these scientists kitted out with all their gadgets, often of their own making, were their playgrounds. They studied the essential nature of light, electricity and magnetism. The combinations of the musing of the intellect with the rock-hard demands of unforgiving science, with its requirements of concrete experiments and reproducible results, brought forth the quantum theory and its mechanics.

With steady inexorable progress, this led them to grasp the underlying nature of matter, the universe, and the role human consciousness played in it. They could hardly believe what they had discovered. The closest mankind had ever come to reaching such depth of understanding was through the ancient meditation trances of Buddhist monks. Also in contradistinction to the West, with its emphasis on development of understanding about the truth of matter's essence being shared throughout its society, the East developed its own take on exploration.

Unlike a common misperception that the East is mankind's locus of mass conformity group think, the Zen Buddhists evolved a form of questioning that was left to the *individual* to answer. Thus knowledge was advanced within each acolyte's own brain as the master monks used Aristotle-style questioning to help the student advance in individual enlightenment. Sometimes this took the from of a poem, as in the Japanese koan, a riddle with possible different answers that developed intuitive thinking.

Furthermore, whilst the East still relied heavily on the meditative approach to understanding, with the stilled quiet mind, or samatha, the West added one more powerful tool to their armamentarium. Work. Action followed their ideas. The English language contains more *verbs*, symbolically denoting action, than say the Chinese language, which contains more nouns, reflecting a respect for a more passive, durable stability, avoiding rapid change. The stress on action and work is the final step of your self-help book's teachings.

This cardinal and seminal difference with the East's emphasis on passive meditation and achieving a still, almost stoned-out mind, and the West's diligent, never-ceasing Calvinistic work ethic, accelerated progress and was celebrated by such scientists of the Faraday cage invention, and the discovery of electromagnetic rotation found in your electric motors today.

"The five essential entrepreneurial skills for success are, concentration, discrimination, organization, innovation and communication."
—Michael Faraday, physicist

The role of action, and specifically work, cannot ever be ignored in your quest for self-improvement. Although this commonplace common sense is sometimes casually shrugged of in modern self-help books, it is essential and necessary for achievement, and it is something all of us can do.

> *"No one can arrive from being talented alone,*
> *work transforms talent into genius."*
> —Anna Pavlova, ballerina

Ironically, after replacing the formal Newtonian classical physics for the subatomic world with the quantum theory and mechanics of Bohr and Heisenberg, it dawned on them that the standard scientific research model of "hypothesis, experiment, results, correct hypothesis, and repeat" cycle, with all the work and effort that entailed, was in serious trouble.

In acknowledging that our human thought either jinxed or actually drove the experimental results, the "Copenhagen Interpretation" dodged the responsibility of handling and defining what observation actually was. They just up and quit using the very scientific method that had brought them thus far. Judge the meaning of the Copenhagen Interpretation for yourself:

> *"At moments of OBSERVATION a different process takes over,*
> *a DIRECT INTERACTION BETWEEN HUMAN*
> *CONSCIOUSNESS AND SUBATOMIC PHYSICS.*
> *One particular state of consciousness becomes real, the rest*
> *were only possibilities."*

Furthermore, the Copenhagen Interpretation of this "alleged" process of *observation* specified a fuller description of *observation*, deemed "a task for the future" or "perhaps forever beyond human comprehension."

These superb and great minds copped out, overwhelmed by the reality of what they had uncovered. In an astonishing, but revealing admission of the unreality of what his experimental apparatus contained, the very progenitor of the Quantum Theory repeatedly stressed to all who would listen, that his results were surreal:

"The quantum world does not exist."
—Niels Bohr

So the stage was set for explanations to fill this great hole. Physicists scoured the globe and stumbled upon the mystic writings of the East. Their very obscurity permitted loose comparisons and adoption into the fold of quantum explanations of matter's essence, and by extension us, our minds, and the universe. Books were written attempting to enfold the ancient wisdom of the East into the inexplicable discoveries of Western science.

Overreach crept in, and Eastern mysticism was accepted whole-sale by some, cramming in disparate, uncritical, incompatible ideas and cultural mores into a one-size-fits-all philosophical box. This persists to the present day, with some self-help books extolling the virtues of the mystic's world to the exclusion of western values that have created so much good for civilization, often blurring the line between wishful thinking and practical pragmatic western reality.

Two oversimplified examples, the American road trip, and sports, may cement this realization, that the fact of being human of necessity includes some of our nasty animal traits. Without which we would nothing more than the lifeless artificial intelligence (AI) computers of the mathematicians, who for the life of them cannot figure out why their AI machines can't think and be motivated like us bipedal dunces. The answer why this is so is outlined below.

Analogies are always intrinsically flawed, but if you can, imagine if you will two cars on a classic American road trip crossing our glorious West. One carries two Buddhist monks seeking samatha, satori and nirvana in a rural setting. The other car has your typical American family setting off on a traditional road trip. After leaving town the Buddhists reach a nice viewpoint on a secluded pullout, displaying some pristine snow-capped mountains. They exit the car, settle comfortably in their yoga lotus positions and begin their meditations and veg out.

Whizzing past them is the boisterous American family, gobbling up the awesome scenery, always wanting more, always seeking the spectacular, energized by desires seeping up from the limbic cellar of their brains, juicing them up. Their passions, given free rein, are hell-bent intent on moving on, forever exploring the wonders of the new and different. Eager to see what's over the next rise, they drive on in the comforting knowledge they can pull over almost any time to chill out in a convenient motel's air conditioning or dunk in its swimming pool. They are driven by deep urges and spirit, with a need to wander and discover what is fresh and new, fueled by the emotions welling up from within their heads, rising up from their limbic systems, the passion center of their brains.

Sport is an American passion. It would not exist without the limbic system. The proxy battles of surrogate warriors on the football field depend on aggression, occasional bursts of fear and anger: in short, our emotions. Fans roar and cheer the combatants, urging on their tribe to make the kill, score that goal. The fans' bubbling enthusiasm is reflected in their gladiatorial champions' ability to earn over fifteen million dollars a year, so great is the extended advertising audience for this tribal battle.

All this energy, this power, and yes, this wealth, derives from the motivational impulses of the limbic system, once called our reptilian brain, not the logic circuits of the cerebral cortex. Unfortunately, the selfsame limbic impulses spawn the murder and mayhem of your daily news, movies and paperback novels. Curiosity, an urge to dominate, seeking power, and rage, sparked by the limbic system's hormones, fueled mankind's wars of conquest and his great explorations of our planet, his visits to the moon, and soon, Mars. We undoubtedly will, and must, populate our Milky Way galaxy if we are to escape engulfment of our lovely earth by the dying sun five billion years hence. It is who we are, we humans. Without a computational limbic system to juice the works, the Artificial Intelligence crowd will never, ever, create a computer that thinks like us.

"People who lean on logic and philosophy and rational exposition, end by starving the best part of the mind."
—William Butler Yeats, poet

It also provides impetus and passion for laughter, encoding the social taboos so freely violated in the best of humor. Without humor how else could man survive the absurd, asinine reality that he is living in the middle of nowhere, on a bunch of rock hurtling through space at 67,000 miles per hour, around a monstrous ball of nuclear explosions, with the total, irrevocable and absolute knowledge that he is going to die?

Yet, and this may seem as heresy to some, Buddhism in its search for samatha, or peaceful tranquility, is a negation of the limbic system, a denial of our humanity. Perhaps suppression, control, dissipation or overriding of the limbic system would reflect its goal more accurately. The end result is the same. Samathic meditation's stated goal is to be goal-less, without need, to suppress appetites, distract us from carnal desires, and to dispel the energies welling up from our limbic system. This abnegates the vital urges that make us for better or worse human, and have driven civilization upward out of the caves into a world of promising continued prosperity. Without desire, your self-help book is useless scrap paper.

This is a harsh critique. Most Buddhist practitioners exude a benevolent love and warmth of their fellow man, and wish nothing more than happiness for all. And they are right: our limbic system is the direct cause of much human suffering, wars, murder and miseries. It should get with the program and fly right.

Nevertheless, we are goal-seekers. We enjoy the suffuse feeling of mastery in what some term the "flow" of practicing a well-honed skill achieving perfect results, on the stage, in the workshop, art studio or kitchen. Work at its best, rejoicing our self-expression, made us what we are today. Work provides a fulfillment that no other endeavor can approach, so addictive to some, and embodied into the matrix of America's exceptionalism, which permits and encourages this form of self affirmation.

Withdrawal into the mind, whilst soothing troubled psyches and providing insightful answers for some, provides no permanent solutions or joy to humankind. This American exceptionalism, recognizing that power is inherent in each individual, with its jubilation and exultation of work, has been encouraged and celebrated by many of its thoughtful leaders.

> *"Far and away the best prize life has to offer*
> *is the chance to work hard at work worth doing."*
> —Theodore Roosevelt

Earlier self-help books stressed this ethos, with the necessity of planning and working of your plan until executed.

> *"If you fail to plan, you're planning to fail."*
> —Anonymous proverb

More recent self-help books slack off and dislocate this connection between your imaginative thoughts, putting your plan to work, then enjoying working your plan for results. Work or action is necessary. It cannot be ignored. You cannot, as some self-help books now suggest and insist, rely solely on thinking the right thoughts for your wealth and desires to suddenly reach fruition. If nothing else, work is a good insurance policy against failures of miraculous manifestation without any action on your part.

Of course, this must be tempered with your constantly held positive vision, for if the physicists are correct with their assessment of time in the multiverse, your vision is already extant, just waiting for your constant thought to dissolve away all your other life path possibilities.

"All that we are is the result of our thoughts.
With our thoughts we make the universe."
—Buddha

CHAPTER THIRTEEN

FEAR, NEGATIVE EMOTIONS
AND MOTIVATION

Your self-help book rightly teaches awareness of your thoughts and feelings, especially negative ones, if only to sustain your mental health, but primarily to free your sensorium to dwell on the results you want. So these pesky, unpleasant nasties can be put to use in spite of all that? Yes, they can.

So, if we fire up our limbic system by fostering solely negative emotions such as fear and anxiety, they will certainly providing us with juice, but are not places we want to stay at. Anxiety or fear does provocatively energize you to seek answers, then persist against obstacles. The Navy SEALS, who certainly could be excused from harboring negative emotions such as well-warranted fear, train under the maxim:

"Scared? You should be. But that's just your body's way of saying it's alive. Now go to work."
—SEALS Training Manual Cannon & Cannon

The more scary and terrorizing your anxiety-provoking goals may be, the more successful they can be.

"Absurd aspirations often lead to unexpected success"
—Churchill

So the negative nasty heebie-jeebies can be useful at times, but persistent and more healthful positive emotions will undoubtedly help you keep going longer without subjecting your body to the risk of chronic diseases brought on by all that retained negativity.

A cookbook list of instructions could include the basics, such as thought awareness with instant recognition of any downer thought nagging you. Your cookbook response would be immediate supplantation and substitution with a positive affirmation, preferably beginning with the powerful "I AM…"As an example, when faced with a pile of bills, or your sales are dropping like a stone, recognize this, then substitute "I am getting better and better. I am turning things around." As cornball as this sounds, it truly does alter your mindset with enough repetition.

The old Indian parable helps illuminate this process and your personal responsibility to monitor your self-talk and correct your negatives. The story goes that a wise old Indian chief comes across an angry young Indian brave, who is cussing about his stolen pony. Even in his angst, the young man is smart enough to seek help and asks the wise elder for guidance. After some thought and reflection, the chief explains: "You have two wolves fighting in your head. The first wolf is vengeful, full of anger, justification, fear, sorrow, doubt, worry, self-pity and unworthiness. The second wolf is brimming with joy, harmony, love, growth, confidence, forgiveness, power, optimism, courage and trust."

After pondering on these words for awhile, the young brave questions the chief again. "But which wolf will win the fight?"

The chief's answer now is immediate: "It depends which wolf you feed."

And so it is. Our retained thoughts are our choice. As our fortieth US president observed:

"Optimism is a choice, and one of the most powerful we can make."
—Ronald Reagan

Many of us muddle through life day to day without really asking the question: "What do I really want?" and, with that omission, sacrifice motivation. Self-help books demand that you confront this question, fully aware that your answers fire up your motivation. When, in your own words, with your brain listening, you begin to articulate your goals alongside new targets and dreams, your subconscious hears you, and activates your RAS, stimulating focus and attention to environmental cues that will inspire and incentivize you.

Thus spurred on, your creativity kicks in and you create maps or stepwise programs to sate your nagging subconscious prompts. Action, in the direction of your goals, is an extremely important modifier and reinforcer of your thoughts. Your action brings conviction, and imprints the belief and trust that your goal is indeed achievable. Your ego now identifies with your project as part of the definition of you, creating the courage and energy necessary for you to persist. The quality of persistence is hammered home repeatedly in your self-help books, because you will face obstacles that have to be overcome.

> *"Nothing in the world can take the place of Persistence.*
> *Talent will not; nothing is more common than unsuccessful men*
> *with talent. Genius will not; unrewarded genius is almost a proverb.*
> *Education will not; the world is full of educated derelicts. Persistence*
> *and determination alone are omnipotent. The slogan 'Press On'*
> *has solved and always will solve the problems of the human race."*
> —Calvin Coolidge

You may be thinking "Well, this is just plain common sense," and you would be right. However, it is amazing that when a person is suffering and wretched about their life's situation, yet makes the effort to pick up a self-help book, just how refreshing and supportive this advice can be. Once out of their mental rut, these work-ethic-worthy tools require no dalliance in the world of the supernatural, nor metaphysical miracles to begin their road to recovery.

Ridding yourself of negative thoughts and their sycophant emotions allows the gloom and doom to lift, with an influx of joy and happiness. Again and again, your self-help book proclaims the cardinal need to be happy, with the attendant feelings of positive optimism and confidence that things will get better, are all of one piece, integral to goal pursuit and achievement. Here comes that new job and car!

Even with a modicum of fear, relaxed optimism and emoting joy help fuel the courage to take a calculated risk and act.

"In playing ball, or in life, a person occasionally gets the opportunity to do something great. When that time comes, only two things matter: being prepared to seize the moment and having the courage to take your best swing."
—Hank Aaron, baseball player

In the face of cancer, patients who can focus their thoughts on relaxation improve their results with chemotherapy dramatically, with fewer side effects and quicker remissions. Just replacing the thoughts of your gym workout from sheer drudgery to a haven as your own personal energy booster can make your performance run smoother and stronger, with precise positive language creating the shift.

Exerting our will on the universe may be a uniquely human characteristic that *in extremis* may alter its very evolution. That's some responsibility!

Shakespeare extolled us to keep our nerve as in his doubts speech:

"our doubts are traitors,
and make us lose the good,
we oft might win,
by fearing to attempt."

Fear was a frequent cockpit companion to the female flier, Amelia Earhart, who faced up to it with her courageous maxim:

"Fears are paper tigers that dissolve when confronted.
Tenacity is all that is then needed to complete the job."
—Amelia Earhart, flier

Fear is definitely an unwelcome visitor to your comfort zone. Yet it remains one of man's most powerful motivators as pointed out by many commentators through the ages.

"Depend on it sir, when a man knows he is to be hanged in a
fortnight, it concentrates his mind wonderfully."
—Samuel Johnson

All the drama and struggle we associate with fear involves our coming to grips with it, persisting, as championed by that old warrior who loved the challenge of the fight:

"Never, never, never, never give in."
—Churchill

It is the trade-offs, the realistic compromises that give zest to life even under the most brutal, dastardly threats and circumstances. Motivation comes in many forms.

"I'll make him an offer he can't refuse."
—Don Corleone, played by Marlon Brando in *The Godfather*

A sense of purpose is essential for you to combat your fears and develop an ability, forbearance, to live through them hour by hour day by day, until it becomes habitual, like all the other new traits that you are seeking with your self-help studies.

"The chains of habit are too weak to be felt until they are too strong
to be broken."
—Samuel Johnson

Lifting the curtain of your comfort zone creates anxieties and fears as your ego fights the change your intellect is seeking. Fear is suppressed by expressing gratitude. The flood of warmth and confidence from gratitude, so repeatedly stressed in your self-help guide, is one of the best, most powerful, antidotes to fear. Say "Thank you" for all your current blessings, no matter how seemingly insignificant, nor how far away from your dreams. This flood of warmth probably reflects a surge of the neurotransmitters dopamine, serotonin and others hitting the rewards centers in your pre-frontal cortex. Nature's very own self-help machine.And it is your dreams and goals that determine your expectations, as you give thanks along the way for life's gifts to you. The dreams you focus on determine what you believe, which in turn define expected results.

> *"Dream as if you'll live for ever, live as if you'll die today."*
> —James Dean, actor

Without purpose dreams or goals you are worse than rudderless before the gales of life's stormy seas; you will lack motivation. Your work, your job, as your self-help loudly proclaims, is to ascertain what it you really want and make choices.

> *"When a man does not know which harbor he is making for,*
> *no wind is the right wind."*
> —Seneca, Roman writer

Or in the words of that great baseball philosopher:

> *"You've got to be very careful if you don't know where you're going,*
> *because you might not get there."*
> —Yogi Berra

Scorn from others hurts your pride and self-esteem. This, although negative, is a strong motivator as you seek to avoid shame.

> *"A useless life is an early death."*
> —Goethe

Dripping with caustic, sardonic, contemptuous malice, the social sages pile on the lash to excoriate those of us who choose to live without purpose and suffer motivational lack. They suggest the ultimate penalty, contradicting their own liberal ethos with a fascistic bent, for those with the asperity to ignore motivational need.

"We should all be obliged to appear before a board every five years and justify our existence...on pain of liquidation."
—George Bernard Shaw, playwright

Your self-help advises you to stay happy, and some of our motivators resort to the humorous twist to raise that wry smile on our faces, in their attempts to light-heartedly remind us what our real purpose on this earth is.

"We are here on earth to do good for others.
What the others are here for I don't know."
—W. H. Auden, writer

Or as we expand on in the final chapter, we can muse the wisdom of a world champion boxer on self-motivation through a sense of purpose.

"Service to others is the rent you pay for your room here on earth."
—Muhammed Ali

CHAPTER FOURTEEN

SUMMATION AND QUERIES

"First, do no harm."
—Hippocratic oath (modern)

When caring for patients, one of the first lessons for a doctor is to not worsen the patient's condition through one's treatment. The second admonition is "to comfort always." Scientists learn the ability to hold two or more, often competing and perhaps contradictory, hypotheses in their minds, and that it is important to factually back up all their assertions whilst retaining the facts of opposing views, should fresh evidence dispute their own pet thesis. Hence, scientists can make maddeningly frustrating talk-show guests, with their infuriating "but on the other hand" arguments as they attempt to do justice to both points of view. As both a former scientist, and now a doctor, my attempt to bring some understanding to the claims of your self-help book borrows some obligation from both these vantage points. This is well illustrated with the expression of two opposing scientific viewpoints on the significance or lack thereof, of humanity's lot in the universe, by one of my heroes:

"Two possibilities exist: either we are alone in the universe, or we are not. Both are equally terrifying."
—Arthur C. Clarke

One of the most intriguing, yet disconcerting aspects of your self-help books, is that almost all the authors state a belief in the metaphysical, paranormal nature of our unconscious mind. This part of our brain's work, the subconscious, carries on about ninety-nine percent or more of our mental activity, with our conscious mind unknowing and uncaring as to its automatic function in keeping our bodies and brains running smoothly.

An additional step is taken, stridently by some, that our subconscious projects out from our bodies and engages and interacts with the universe, which is pictured as embodying a universal mind or energy field in cahoots with our brains and our wishes. Dragooned into this mix is the noble scientific arena of quantum theory and mechanics, wed to their self-help theories in a sometimes unwilling shotgun marriage. Long on conjecture, but short on proof, this subconscious-universe link is an abiding theme present in most self-help treatises. The key issues revolve around the spicy (and best-selling) proposition that human will and thought can communicate outside the brain with the universe and affect future events in one's life in a positive fashion. Fantastic metaphysics if true, demanding full attention of all the hard-nosed scientists and re-structuring the education of our children.

There is certainly enough confusion, contradiction and (pun intended) uncertainty in the genesis of the quantum theory to provide grounds for both the scrupulous and the charlatan to mix it with all the unknowns and unknowables of the nature of human consciousness to provide a rich feast for the metaphysical zealot. Even the sober layperson cannot readily refute or easily comprehend claims made about the meshing of quantum physics with the workings of his mind. Indeed, this book itself has put its toe in this water, permitted opposing or inconsistent statements, attempted to deliberately escape the editor's scouring and censorial pen, examined and provoked such possibilities, and danced with paranormal explanations. Unashamedly so, because answers are lacking, much work remains, both in neurobiology and in physics. This is not an abdication of responsibility brought on by my schizophrenic career constraints, but a real desire to explore with you, the reader, evolving thoughts on the validity of a mind-universe connection. The answers are not yet in. Is quantum theory to blame for this mess? Do the physicists know the biology?

Translating thoughts into words using electrodes on the head is a real fact, called brain reading. Thoughts are indeed real things, as your self-help book proclaims. Just thinking a word, such as "hungry," without verbalization, is enough for electrodes to pick up and identify the correct word with appropriate electronics. "Hungry" shows up on a computer screen. Amazing stuff that will undoubtedly help stroke victims. Other research shows that paraplegics, appropriately monitored, just asked to think about moving a limb, can have these thoughts detected, monitored and used to signal an external motor to move their paralyzed arms in the correct visualized direction. Brain waves can synchronize between couples eliciting similar thoughts and words, in a biological, proven, natural fashion demolishing a once-paranormal sixth sense conjecture. This is powerful stuff and cannot be fobbed off as hyperbole used to market self-help books. Is there is more to thought projection than just signaling locally?

Physicists make the sound argument that quantum events occur now in the universe where no humans exist, and will continue in the universe long after the human race has left the scene, and all consciousness snuffed with its departure, thus demolishing the claim that quantum events are dependent on human conscious thought.

Likewise, the concept of a universal aether permeating the universe has been categorically shown not to exist by a long series of exquisitely careful light experiments. This challenges the self-help book contention of an all-pervading supraconscious energy field united with the matter of the universe, something self-help books joyously and freely claim without bothering to verify with evidence.

Physicists mock this as unwarranted narcissism on the part of a self-absorbed humanity whose miniscule and insignificant presence in the vastness of the universe's size and age is inconsequentially trivial. Remember that voice on the Discovery Channel?

"Billions upon billions of stars!.
—Carl Sagan

The fault, if any, lies at the start of the quantum theory, with its deliberate avoidance of naming observers, and defining observation in the Copenhagen Interpretation. Bohr and Heisenberg were brilliant and sincere when they volunteered that perhaps explaining that their experimental findings was "a task for the future, or perhaps forever beyond human comprehension." They dropped the ball in not pursuing this, as the quantum theory worked so well at making other predictions, so they just ran with that.

As a long-suffering father, I would reprimand and chastise my young daughter for some idleness or slacking off with the old-fogey line "when I was a lad we used to walk five miles in the sleet and snow…. to wherever" (and I am sure those of my generation can finish this sentence themselves in hundreds of ways, because we all heard it countless times from our own parents). In the insouciance of disrespectful youth, her cheeky response would always be: "Dad, that was then; this is now!" This always settled the argument in her favor. You never win. And so it is with physics.

That was then. This is now. Physics, especially quantum physics, has learned and evolved. The weasel words, anomalies and conundrum of the Copenhagen Interpretation, used so triumphantly by the new agers to insinuate their one-conscious-mind-energy-field-combo-universe into physics, have been put to rest by advances in the science. Or so the physicists tell us in their obscure and almost impenetrable work, with no thought to the lay person's attempt to understand with all the good will and effort in the world. And these guys live off research grants, so their PR efforts need a little enhancement. Einstein at his jovial best noted that scientific research, though great fun, was no way to make a living. Having been there in my former life, I concur.

Dumbfoundedly, with all sincerity and assurance from research findings and new theories on multiple universes, leading physicists claim the observer conundrum is dismissed with the utterly banal explanation that if the progenitors of the Copenhagen Interpretation had just used the word "instrument" instead of "observers" and the act of "observation" then this whole mystery would never have arisen. Judge the language for yourself.

> *"If Bohr and Heisenberg had spoken of measurements made*
> *by inanimate instruments rather than 'observers' perhaps the*
> *strained relationship between quantum and mind would not*
> *have been drawn. For nothing in quantum mechanics require*
> *human intervention."*
> —Victor J. Stenger, quantum physicist

The mysterious effects at a distance of entangled particles, which show instantaneous correlation when one measures the property of the first subatomic particle, is a coincident effect that is determined in its matched particle, up to ten miles away. These experiments, which measure properties such as particle spin, have been repeated many times with unequivocal results. The conundrum arises because this nonlocality suggests signaling faster than the speed of light, or superluminal, which is forbidden in Einstein's relativity. The way out of this is to step back and get to a higher level, as when we were crossing that river in the earlier chapter. What the physicist did was to correct their language and thus their thinking. Looking at the things which were being measured, they asked themselves: What are these characteristics we measure? Are they real solid entities, or are they just a bunch of fancy sums? And so they found their escape route. They called what they were measuring "mathematical constructions," and thus relieved them of the duty to be receiving signals. The quandary of superluminal signals, moving faster than the speed of light, and a mainstay of the metaphysical paranormal ideology, just evaporated. The mathematical constructions were described in lay terms as just vectors or geometrical shapes. Well, that sorts that lot out once and for all, doesn't it?

Just to pound that into all those thick skulls the physicists let loose:

> *"What we perceive, determine, or even control what is out there, is without rational foundation."*
> —Victor J. Stenger, quantum physicist

And in case you missed the point:

> *"Quantum consciousness is a myth, along with gods, unicorns, and dragons."*
> —Victor J. Stenger, quantum physicist

This "mathematical creations of our imagination" explanation was extended to the enigmatic "particle versus wave duality." In this evolution of ideas, the only thing that is superluminal, moving faster than the speed of light, is just a mentally created bunch of sums. This included the quantum wave function, which did not collapse into that particle that popped up like an unwanted guest at a party from the void, but was just a reflection of how you set up your instrument to detect it. One instrumental set-up gets you a wave, another gets you a particle. That's all there is to it, so get over it.

Well, the Oracle has spoken and we mere mortals must accept its judgment. Your self-help book's foray into the quantum world in search of a paranormal metaphysical dimension appears to be shriveling under the counterattack from the guys who write the physics textbooks. Is this deliberate deception? Or do the self-help authors all believe it?

The paranormal worldview keeps shrinking. This dismissal of superluminal signaling is a deal-breaker. The discovery that the sixth sense of spouses knowing each others' thoughts has been ascribed to nothing more than synchronization of each others' brain waves is fun stuff, but still falls under the scope of regular old biology. The much-trumpeted "out of body" experience near death is just your right angular gyrus on the blink, needing a service call.

The Buddhist monk's "oneness with the universe" is just a dissociation from self-induced shut down of the OAA brain system. The tunnel with a central bright light as you begin to check out: just your occipital cortex vision center running out of oxygen, blotting out your peripheral vision. It happens to fighter pilots pulling G's shutting down blood circulation to their occiputs all the time. Enlightenment of the Veda mystic, Sanskrit poetry scriptures, all helped along the way with hits of ecstasy-like ephedrine.

This list continues to grow, like ghost stories on Halloween that disappear when the sun comes up to shine brightly the next morning. Unexplained superstitions, all of them, but is that totally true? Are there those niggling little exceptions that defy explanation and upset our perfectly arranged display on the applecart?

Let us revisit that poor old Scots soldier, William Murray's, escape from certain death whilst under Jerry bombardment, and my own dream of Dad pointing to his metastatic cancer pain in his back. What do they have in common, and what can we explain away in light of modern biology?

Both experiences were extremely intense, all consuming, vivid, totally unique to the individual, never again experienced, once-in-a-lifetime events during stress. Of finite time and duration, information of extreme importance was raised to the level of acute conscious awareness in both people. Murray's experience could be explained away as an almost caricature of a cartoonish message from God booming out his life-saving warning. Readers of this book are not so intellectually lazy to hide in ignorance, with such an indolent cop-out, and not seek out the factual causes involved.

Differences abound. Murray's overwhelming brain attack was

totally aural, a loud voice, with the powerful intense command, "Stay still. Don't move!" No visuals.

Let us analyze further. You don't have to be an Inspector Clouseau, or even a doctor, to recognize a few salient clues. Murray was wired, he was in battle, involved in intense combat. His blood adrenaline level must have been through the roof. He had just experienced the trauma of seeing his dispatch runner shot in two with his legs still running around, like the proverbial chicken with its head cut off.

Moreover, Murray himself had just lived through the shell explosion that created the crater next to him. His body fluids were still absorbing the shock waves. His brain was concussed. His hearing was temporarily deadened from the noise of the blast. The shock of all this would have jacked up his adrenaline to off-the-chart levels. His vision would be temporarily blinded from the intense light of the explosion. His two major senses, sight and vision, were temporarily severely compromised or nearly shut down.

The dream I experienced was intense, vivid, entirely visual, repetitive in real time, involved a dear relative in acute distress, and contained highly relevant information. No prompts or cues, subtle or otherwise, preceded the exact detailed nature of the dream. No drugs were ingested. Sleep pattern was normal. Yet there it was, over and over, prompting unusual action in me the next morning. It was intense, unsubtle, unforgettable, like getting hit with a two-by-four on the noggin.

My body does not take well to having foreign proteins from a horse injected into it. As a teenager with a broken arm from falling off my push-bike I landed in the county hospital. I was given a tetanus shot cooked up in horse serum. My body did not like it. As my trachea went into laryngospasm, choking off my airway, and the shades began closing in, the grim reaper joined the party in the corner of the room, musing it was a little early to collect a young soul, but he'd take what he could get.

Fortunately for me, a young nurse came into the waiting room and recognized my plight. She stuck a syringe in my arm and pumped me full of adrenaline. Immediately the trachea relaxed. I could breathe again. Oxygen flooded my brain, along with a bolus of that adrenaline. What a rush, vivid, intense, bright, alive, wired, feeling like a million bucks, omnipotent.

It is that level of intensity that Murray must have felt with his aural hallucination, and I certainly felt that way with the dream. Biology dictates that everything we experience in our sensorium must originate within our brains. Natural, non-paranormal scientific explanations get the bias. Adrenaline type neurotransmitters are released constantly in very low doses in our brains. Disturbed brains can generate abnormal illusions, particularly when sight is compromised as in sleep, or bleaching of the retinas with explosive bright lights. The mind is used to perceiving stimuli as coming from outside the body, so that when a different part of the brain interprets these chemical disturbances it considers them triggered by external events.

From these horrendous events, learning can sometimes be advanced:

> *"I find hope in the darkest days and focus in the brightest.*
> *I do not judge the universe."*
> —the Dalai Lama

So, as we shrink the paranormal into the normal shoebox of increased understanding, knowledge and hopefully wisdom, how do these events help reveal the secrets of your self-help book? For a start, the less metaphysics you can ascribe to happy coincidences and manifestations of your focused thoughts, the more faith and confidence you will find in yourself to continue your work. Let us attempt to render an analysis of our Scot's lifesaving voice in his head. We have discussed the high adrenaline blood level that must have been flooding his brain. That would impress any interpretation as being intense vivid, loud and clear, perhaps otherworldly.

Schizophrenia has a symptomatic pattern of producing voices inside one's head, along with other hallucinations. Often, brain shrinkage is seen on scans in association with this type of schizophrenia. One of my patients who is a paranoid schizophrenic reports frequently of seeing visions of unreal faces, and when his medication levels get low, hearing voices that the faces are angry at him. With the percussive blast our Scot had just suffered, is it reasonable to conclude that his brain was shaking like a bowl of jelly? Could his auditory hallucination, jacked up with adrenaline, be responsible for his "voice from God?"

Would concussion temporarily upset his brain metabolism so that he lapsed into a brief episode of schizophrenia? Yes is the probable answer to these questions, but what is left out and remains mysterious is the message content itself, which is as of yet inexplicable.

Let us revisit one aspect of the dad dream, before laying out five pointers for those who have experienced similar phenomena, know they are not crazy, and may be a little embarrassed to share with others. Exploring how our brains might work often reveals insights that can help us through obstacles and create fresh goals. Neurobiologists are familiar with recurrent firing patterns in brains, usually cyclical in nature with neurochemical and electrochemical mechanisms available and responsible. Nature at work, nothing metaphysical required. One aspect of the dad dream was the repetitive nature cycling four or five times over. This repetition in my naïve former mind represented a level of importance being given by my brain to its message. That can now be viewed in the light of a natural repetitive firing within the brain, lacking any need for a paranormal explanation.

So let us examine whether these episodes reveal any of the secrets of how your self-help books work, by trying to gain a higher level of perspective as to what is going on without recourse to paranormal excuses. These five steps may be referred to with any future visions that may enter your life without warning, and help you cope with their unsettling nature that most doctors could not explain to your satisfaction.

1. *Adrenaline* Your brain relies on small amounts of adrenergic neurotransmitters such as norepinephrine, which is in the adrenaline family. When elevated, it can create feelings of vivid omnipotency. If such an experience visits you, and you have not ingested any stimulative drugs, ask yourself what excites your mind so much? Is it fear? Is it something of great importance to the survival of your person or people you love?

2. *Entanglement* Couples, friends and families have the chance to share many molecules. Subatomic paired particles can exhibit common mathematical outcomes due to entanglement, when measured in some fashion, and demonstrate this property across large distances. This may exert some influence in an as-yet-undetermined fashion on other people's brains, through the gate switch pores on receptive brain axons as described below.

3. *Gate Switch* The nerve fibers in your brain have switches which can turn them on, existing as special pores which have a trapdoor gate mechanism, guarded by trigger molecules. These trigger molecules can be on or off, acting as a switch, depending upon a quantum superposition of a subatomic particle such as a proton.

If this particle is on one position, the molecular trapdoor lid is closed and the nerve does not fire. If the particle is in the other position, the molecular trapdoor lid opens and the nerve fires. This quantum dependent mechanism could be affected if this key supposition particle is entangled with one outside the head. It could be entangled in another person's brain, or inanimate matter. Whether this mechanism actually operates in human brains has not yet been proven.

At any given time, with the nerves or axons within your head, some are always ready to fire, to have their switches tripped by this proposed mechanism, or other routine mechanisms that normally function in your brain. Amplification of signal can be rapid once one gate pore opens. Other gate pores open on the nerve, increasing signal strength, and other nerves in the vicinity are triggered to fire, creating a signaling surge. A thought or action can then result. All this, from one small change, which can be quantum, in the molecule guarding the gate. This is a natural, highly effective signal amplifier in your brain. A dream or vision could be initiated in this fashion and probably is.

4. *Vision Construction* As discussed in a prior chapter, your vision is created from five or six elements in your retinas, such as vertical line or movement receptors. From this your brain constructs the wonderful awe inspiring panorama of the beautiful outside world all around us. There is no little man watching a movie in your head. It is all a wonderful illusion.

In the dad dream, the visual image was Spartan. It was washed out in color, even whilst being an intense experience. The vividness in felt experience did not carry over into the image. The scene contained few visual elements. Dad in semi-profile, indistinct dark grey background, turned in three-quarter profile, naked to the waist, pointing to the middle of his back, with his arm twisted around to do so. His hair, with face turned in profile, that was about it. It was that cryptic. Little information; however, it entered my head or was created within, was needed to achieve this spare, basic, but highly informative image.

Was some shared brain wave resonating with mine?

5. *Australian Synchronous Brain Waves* The new studies coming out of Australia clearly demonstrate the biological nature of a well-known phenomena between couples. It is exciting and fascinating and may very well indicate what is happening in some cases of self-help manifestations. Couples who have been together for a while often develop the uncanny knack of thinking, then articulating the

same thoughts simultaneously. My spouse does this from three or four rooms away in the house with alarming frequency.

What the Australian researchers found was that when these phenomena occurred, their measured brain waves were in synchrony. It appears that what poor old Carl Jung lacked to prove his theories of synchronicity was an appropriate instrument for measuring brain waves! The researchers have not published the maximum distance separating the couples who could synchronize their brain waves, and this will be of intense interest to the current discussion.

Synchronization of brain waves is a form of resonance. Resonance occurs in the classic example of the sound waves from the fat lady of the opera singing her high notes. When these waves resonate at the appropriate frequency in a crystal glass, it shatters. Similarly, on a much larger scale, the earthquake off Sumatra that caused devastating tsunamis which drowned thousands of victims was reported by geologists to cause the entire planet, in their words, to "ring like a bell." Some resonance!

So as we shred the last vestige of the paranormal from the dad dream, and reclaim our scientific sanity and pride, we must query, was this resonance? Six thousand miles away? Was the dad dream resonant, in synch brain waves? Hardly the "good vibrations" of the old Beach Boys song, but you get the picture.

So what about the content conundrum, if we do away with the need for superluminal signal transmission, with a large data dump packet, how would resonance work with dad pointing to his back? Well, as we have taken a step back from the quantum and the need for a universal mind, by invoking a different mechanism that of brain wave resonance, let us back up a bit further, and throw in two additional facts drawn from my family's combined medical experience.

My elder sister is a trained clinical psychologist, which is annoying enough to begin with, and although she vigorously denies it, she allows that supercilious superiority of being my older sister peek through the veneer of her professional demeanor. So when I reviewed the dad dream with her some while back, her first response was not the expected fascination of curiosity, but her irritating retreat into professional clinical psychologese, "Well, what did it *mean* to you?" "Well Sis, it meant Dad was pointing to his painful back and I somehow locked into that channel because he wanted to communicate that with me."

Wrong answer. Wrong meaning, because my interpretation was incorrect. Read on, and I'll let you solve this riddle, see the now obvious misinterpretation, and then you may apply it to your own dreams.

My wife is a nurse who has treated cancer patients in extreme distress in the ICU of cancer wards at a large cancer research hospital. My early years saw me working as a PhD cancer research scientist at the same institute, then later I became a medical doctor treating live patients, not rats. Let me assure that these combined experiences have taught us both that metastatic bone pain can be excruciatingly painful and difficult to treat.

Now, for all you budding detectives out there, my next question is: what do you do when part of your body is in pain? That's right, Sherlock, you *rub* it.

If, as I now suspect, Dad was in such agony as to even think about going to a hospital, let alone admitted, he was in some pretty serious pain. Again, let me share a doctor's perspective about patients in severe pain. They regress. They fold in on themselves, fixated on their pain, its history, what it feels like to touch, what it takes to rub away and ameliorate that nagging discomfort. It consumes them, all their waking hours, until relief can be provided. It occupies all their thoughts in a singular attempt to understand it. They obsess about it with the emotional intensity your self-help book advises when you wish to manifest something. Your pain becomes your entire mental world. And you constantly try to rub it away.

Now let us return to the Australian model of synchronized brain waves between loved ones. There is no attempt to communicate. Communication is inherent in the brain wave synchrony. Dad responded to my queries that no, he had not thought of me, just his back pain. By now you have figured this out, where there line of reasoning is leading. What I actually saw was *dad's fingers on his back*. What I interpreted it as was *pointing*. What he was actually doing was *rubbing*.

This distinction is critically important. The real action, back *rubbing,* is a solitary image, infused and highly charged with pain energy though it may be passive with regards to signaling, and does not require, infer or impose a will to communicate. In contrast, back *pointing* implies an active attempt to communicate with another person, open to my egocentric interpretation as an implied receiver of a telepathic signal, but reflecting a desire, will and ability to communicate between two people.

My error reflected an attempt of analysis that involved psychic communication from an active sender (Dad) to a recipient (me) using superluminal quantum signaling. The facts did not fit. Dad had no recollection of even thinking about me, he could not have been an active sender. In my defense of this *mea culpa*, the resonance of brain waves was unknown to me or anyone else at the time at my initial attempts at analysis.

Injunction of the paranormal was not necessary. My natural scientific skepticism was overridden by the intense personal emotional events resulting in my father's death. It should be an object lesson for others working through emotional stress. Trying so valiantly to think through a problem without sufficient firepower from accurate knowledge is a recipe for gullibility. It is small consolation that many others of far greater intellect than I have been blindsided with similar self-deception.

This is a mistake you the reader might make, and should thus be aware of if you share similar experiences, of trying to shoehorn available facts into whatever model of the quantum universal mind you have picked up from your self-help books. Don't allow yourself to be misled in fields of which you have little training or knowledge. It can take a long time to dig out from laboring under such delusions. No matter how intense and honestly held the beliefs of the authors of these tomes may be, it does not assure you that they are correct. Hence my first admonition to the self-help authors is that line from our doctor's modern Hippocratic oath: "First, do no harm."

> *"Our prime purpose in life is to help others.*
> *And if you can't do that, at least don't hurt them."*
> —the Dalai Lama

To wrap this up, let me paint you a picture with an analogy I trust that you will not find too tortured or tedious. My house is blessed with the luxury of an energizing weight work-out room. One of the features of weight-lifting as a form of exercise is that it involves goal setting. Also, of course, it is a constant reminder that you should have skipped that last pint the night before. After laborious years of workouts I finally approached the ability to lift the heaviest weight plate on my machine. This entailed inserting a pin through and under it to secure the weight plate prior to lifting.

It wouldn't fit.

My caveman reaction was to reach for the closest object at hand, a twenty-five-pound barbell, and clobber the pin in. After a couple of sessions doing this, I felt ashamed of myself. Supposedly a smart guy with a bunch of degrees, and hands capable of the most delicate surgeries in the world on eyes and faces, and here I was acting like a chimpanzee, pounding nuts open with a rock.

My good fortune is to have a sophisticated, quick-witted American wife, amongst whose life goals is to maintain me in a permanent state of subservient humility. When in her none too shy, remonstrative, acerbic way she accuses me of primitive, blunt, crude, neanderthalithic, stubborn obstinacy, I readily accede, confess and accept.

Her words echoed through my head as I pounded that weight pin with the iron barbell, with her rebuke from the summers of my English youth, working the fields of the farms in Lancashire, "You can take the boy out of the farm, but you can't take the farm out of the boy!"

So, with one last ape-like grunt, I rose from my simian crouch to examine the problem from a higher level. Sound familiar? Emerging from the top of the stack of weight plates through a small shackle was the weight-lifting steel cable, which penetrated the shackle and weight stack. Curious fingers wiggled the shackle, and voila! The weight holes lined up like tumblers in a lock, and the pin slid home as easy as a hot knife in butter.

Thus, as I pounded away at analysis of the dad dream, using the klutzy barbell of my rudimentary knowledge of neuroscience and my lazy acceptance of the self-help book mantra of universal consciousness field, I was massively frustrated by the abysmal fit, lack of elegance, and the amount of effort involved.

During the early hectic days of building my practice, I was engrossed in slicing open thousands of human eyeballs to restore sight to their owners, and had little time to spare to delve into modern quantum theory. As you have learned if you have had the patience to stick with the story so far, I paid for that idleness in spades.

When growing up near Liverpool, one of the hyperboles of the scouser street toughs during my nighttime forays downtown was that if I crossed them they would "rearrange my face." In an ironic twist, after a trip through the educational meat-grinder, I now make my living as a plastic surgeon, rearranging faces. This type of practice gives me more time to read and explore the intricacies of modern physics.

Hence my acquaintance with the higher levels with which to examine the dad dream mystery. The resonance of human brain waves, demonstrated as real, with the ability to share thoughts and images, is almost a perfect match, like that pin lining up with the weight holes. A much better, more elegant fit, with minimal effort. Yes, problems remain, as my wife reminds me, "Well, six thousand miles is along way to resonate," until I recall the geologists' observation of the Sumatra quake ringing like a bell across the entire surface of the earth. Resonant brain waves sound like so much more fun.

Now that the analysis of the dad dream has been put to bed, can the grownups come out and play with the really scary stuff? Is their even a smidgen of hope for our self-help book's claim to invoke the quantum world in the realization of your dreams? Well, maybe, kinda, sort of. Ironically, it may be that the gurus did not pursue the quantum world avidly enough into its more modern direction. And I may have been a little harsh on the gurus after my own frustrating excursion into their world of universal consciousness.

Perhaps it's time to cut them some slack.

> *"Be kind wherever possible. It is always possible."*
> —the Dalai Lama

The cheeky riposte of my schoolgirl daughter applies to many in the self-help community who are still hung up in the universe-human consciousness time warp—that was then; this is now. The old observer conundrum of now you see it, now you don't of the wave/particle duality is becoming replaced with new mathematics. And it may well be that Einstein's critique, that if you can't explain it then you don't understand it, holds true for the self-help gurus.

When the young Turks in the physics community really pushed the implications of the quantum theory into their own little world of impenetrable mathematics, they came up with a truly scary result. We don't all live in a yellow submarine anymore. Our universe is just one of a gazillion! We live in a multiverse of parallel universes where our self-help books can get up to any kind of nefarious fun, and we can't find them when they play hide and seek.

And multiverse is what the new math requires. In a marvelous twist of bittersweet irony, the very name "multiverse" was coined by none other than that father of the self-help movement, and founder of modern psychology, that quirky, quixotic misfit William James. This is where we need the brilliance of a Jacob Bronowski, to explain all this new annoying real estate in lay terms. This famous physicist was able to lucidly explain man's history and development of science to the great unwashed masses, in the BBC series *The Ascent of Man* in 1975. But your luck, you're stuck with me so I'll keep it brief.

> *"The multiverse is right around you. It arises from random quantum processes that cause the universe to branch into many copies, one for each possible outcome."*
> —Max Tegmark, physicist

The wave function, remember that? It's a math construct that rotates around in a place called Hilbert space which has more dimensions than you could shake a stick at, and then some, and no, I don't have any drugs in my doctor's bag that would help you even dream this stuff up. The old collapse of the wave function, because it was only stupid math after all, now splits into zillions of realities. But the math says you can actually count all of these possibilities, it's a real number, big, but real and determinable, so of course the theory must be correct—got that?

You, as the poor sucker having to watch all this splitting, can now observe it. It is a slight randomness of parallel universes. These can split and merge, giving you any number of story lines. Aha! I smell an opening for the self-help book's multiple story lines; maybe I can live a better one? But you can't see all the copies of yourself living all these different lives like Walter Mitty. Oh no! Decoherence steps in and there is only you left to live in your own little world.

What causes you to split into multiple copies without bleeding all over the damn pavement? Decisions, decisions, decisions. Choices made by your own little mind and the decision to act on them cause the splitting. All your other copies live in that big old Hilbert space, doing what you do where you don't confess. What the hell does all this garbage mean?

"All possible states exist at every instant,
so the passage of time may be in the eye of the beholder."
—Max Tegmark, physicist

It means that everything that is possible becomes real. Time is an illusion, so all these possibilities with you in that new job, new spouse, new car and new home already exist somewhere in these made-up mathematical dimensions. Your self-help books can have a field day with that, and they do. If the physicists are daft enough to give them so much easy fodder then there is no hope of holding the gurus back. You could drive all the world's Mack trucks through the holes in that Hilbert space.

"What's it all about Alfie? Is it just for the moment we live?
What's it all about Alfie, when you sort it out Alfie?".
—David and Bacharach, songwriters

So what's it all about as we reach for our self-help books to climb that greasy pole, assured by now that if we clear our thoughts and visualize with emotion, act when appropriate, we can somehow steer our ship towards the golden shore of our dreams and nudge all these possibilities into existence?

"The trouble with the rat race is that even if you win,
you're still a rat."
—Lily Tomlin, comedienne

Lest you think I belittle the self-help books, contemplate that one of the leading books was written by a surgeon, and I and other surgeons have found, and do find, some of these books of immense help in preparing for surgery, particularly in visualizing good outcomes, and early on, overcoming beginner's jitters, among many other goals.

It is human nature to want more and better for you and yours, so the self-help book will be forever with us, for better or worse.

"The natural effort of every individual to better his own condition is so powerful that it alone, and without any assistance, is not only capable of carrying on the society to wealth and prosperity, but of surmounting one hundred important obstructions with which the folly of human laws too often encumber its operations."
—Adam Smith, *The Wealth of Nations,* 1776

Or, if you prefer the shorter American version of your commitment to hard work on your road to success:

"Everything comes to him who hustles while he waits."
—Thomas Edison

The danger lies in not asking the questions. What if it's all wrong? What if my thoughts will never manifest the way I want? What if that extra copy of me in that next dimension never materializes in my life? How much time have I wasted trying to think that winning Lotto ticket into my sweaty little palm? Shouldn't I have tried to take care of myself using pragmatic steps like getting a new, better-paying job or expanding my old one?

The idea of waiting around till your ship comes in, hoping and praying for that proverbial winning Lotto ticket, is akin to the tragic wasted life of that old maid spinster, put together by my hometown lads, John and Paul:

"Eleanor Rigby ... lives in a dream, waits at the window, wearing the face that she keeps in a jar by the door."
—The Beatles

As this is the chapter of queries, one has to ask. Where is the chapter on work in the self-help books? As Edison and Adam Smith point out, individual effort, working while you wait for your big break, and in the poignancy of Eleanor Rigby waiting at the window for the white knight who never comes to save her, all teach us that nose to the grindstone will at least put bread on your table.

> *"The heights by great men reached and kept,*
> *were not attained by sudden flight,*
> *but they, while their companions slept,*
> *were toiling upward through the night."*
> —Longfellow

This quote I keep above my desk to remind me of those long grueling nights in grad school and my medical training. Reading it always sends an emotional frisson through me. Lacking in almost all the self-help books is that good old American ethic: never let yourself be outworked. This is one of their uglier secrets.

The secret of success for many of the old time captains of industry was necessity, after being thrown out on the street to work around the age of puberty, often due to a parental death or divorce. Finding work, and not spending four years in college, provided many of these winners the need to ascend through their own work efforts. It did not come easy. But when they made it they could look back with pride that they enjoyed their newfound status through their own work, not metaphysics, nor reliance on handouts from others, as framed so long ago by that canny Scot:

> *"It is not from the benevolence of the butcher, the brewer, or the*
> *baker that we expect our dinner, but from their regard to their own*
> *self interest. We address ourselves not to their humanity, but to their*
> *self love, and could never talk to them of our necessities but of their*
> *advantages.".*
> —Adam Smith, *The Wealth of Nations* 1776

In those pre-income tax days these self made men could celebrate their successes with a vengeance. My first step off the boat in America so to speak, was the fun state of Rhode Island. It was here, where I pursued my doctoral studies and landed my first university faculty position in biophysics, that I was able to explore the famed "summer cottages" of the nouveau riche in Newport, Rhode Island. These fabulous rock piles, monuments to excess, fantastic architectural wonders whose likes will never be seen again, adorn the rocky coastline of the Ocean State.

These mansions stand in stark contrast to that other good old American value which is never mentioned in your self-help books. Another ugly secret. Where are the chapters on thrift? Where is the message of prudent husbandry of resources so essential to capital formation? Where is the reflection of that old Yankee pragmatism?

> *"Use it up,*
> *Wear it out,*
> *Make it do,*
> *Or do without."*
> —New England proverb

Modern-day magnates such as Sam Walton of Wal-Mart drove around in a pick-up trick. Sure, his Ford F-150 pick-up truck had all the bells and whistles, but it was still a frugal pickup truck. Warren Buffet, the successful billionaire investor, for many years kept his old, relatively modest home without splurging on excess. Thrift works.

These examples are omitted from the self-help books, and permit daydreaming when real down-to-earth action is required. It is here, in avoiding the values of thrift and hard work necessitating firm choices on your part, that some self-help books violate the maxim to "do no harm."

"Happiness is not something ready made, it comes from your own achievements."
—the Dalai Lama

Ultimately this is about you, and those moments of joy that you can expand, to create the life of your dreams. Your self-help book is a tool to educate you and point the way for you to develop fresh behaviors, resulting in habits that will increase the number of your fulfilling moments.

"Magic moments,
Filled with love."
—Bacharach and David, song *Magic Moments*

Maxwell's equations on electromagnetism opened up the possibility of distant signaling. However, it was Feynman's discovery and insight that particles crossing that famous double slit took every possible path, enjoyed every possible history, even across the universe and back, picking up information, that helped shoulder your self-help book's assertion of universal mind that you could tap into. It's hard to argue with the new quantum physics.

Your self-help book taps into the bizarre underlying reality of time, coupled with the multiple universes brought to us by Everett and expanded upon by Tegmark. Picture our moments as little Facebook video clips, snapshots of your life with every possible history and every possible future. These are all stacked up in a shoebox, way, way too big to fit in the bottom of your closet. They await your selection as to which future you will pick. Your self-help book suggests this happens by your passionate focused thoughts, marinating with the universal mind, when the truth may be far more mundane. Your reticular activating system in your brain alerts you to all the cues necessary, for you to compile choices and personal decisions that will move you towards that desired video clip stuck at the bottom of your shoebox. You turn the steering wheel of your life towards that outcome, and eventually you begin to move in that direction as new opportunities avail themselves.

However, that all being said, there are enough mysteries in the physics of time, and physicists' avowed acceptance that multiple histories and multiple futures all exist contemporaneously, for your self-help books to end up being right after all. We are here, now, in the present moment. This is for you to enjoy. Living your life for some future aspiration takes you out of the now, that will never be revisited in your human time. Enjoy it.

Aphorisms and quotations have been used throughout this book to cement a thought using someone else's perspective on the same topic. You may find the same bubbling enthusiasm, during a stale and plodding day, when a quotation hits just the right note to fire up your synapses, and give you a thread to obsess on as your day unfolds. So I will leave you just one more from a far better trained, kinder, humbler and benevolent mind than mine, which reflects my honest and perhaps clumsy Anglo-Saxon attempts to educate and entertain you. Enjoy the moments!

> *"The purpose of our lives is to be happy."*
> —the Dalai Lama

Lightning Source UK Ltd.
Milton Keynes UK
UKOW050433240412

191341UK00001B/162/P